THE HANDBOOK OF CONSTITUTIONAL AND ENERGETIC HERBAL MEDICINE

THE HANDBOOK OF CONSTITUTIONAL AND ENERGETIC HERBAL MEDICINE
The Lotus Within

Andrew Stableford

AEON

First published in 2020 by
Aeon Books
PO Box 76401
London W5 9RG

Copyright © 2020 by Andrew Stableford

The right of Andrew Stableford to be identified as the author of this work has been asserted in accordance with §§ 77 and 78 of the Copyright Design and Patents Act 1988.

All rights reserved. No part of this publication may be reproduced, stored in a retrieval system, or transmitted, in any form or by any means, electronic, mechanical, photocopying, recording, or otherwise, without the prior written permission of the publisher.

British Library Cataloguing in Publication Data

A C.I.P. for this book is available from the British Library

ISBN-13: 978-1-91280-713-0

Typeset by Medlar Publishing Solutions Pvt Ltd, India
Printed in Great Britain

www.aeonbooks.co.uk

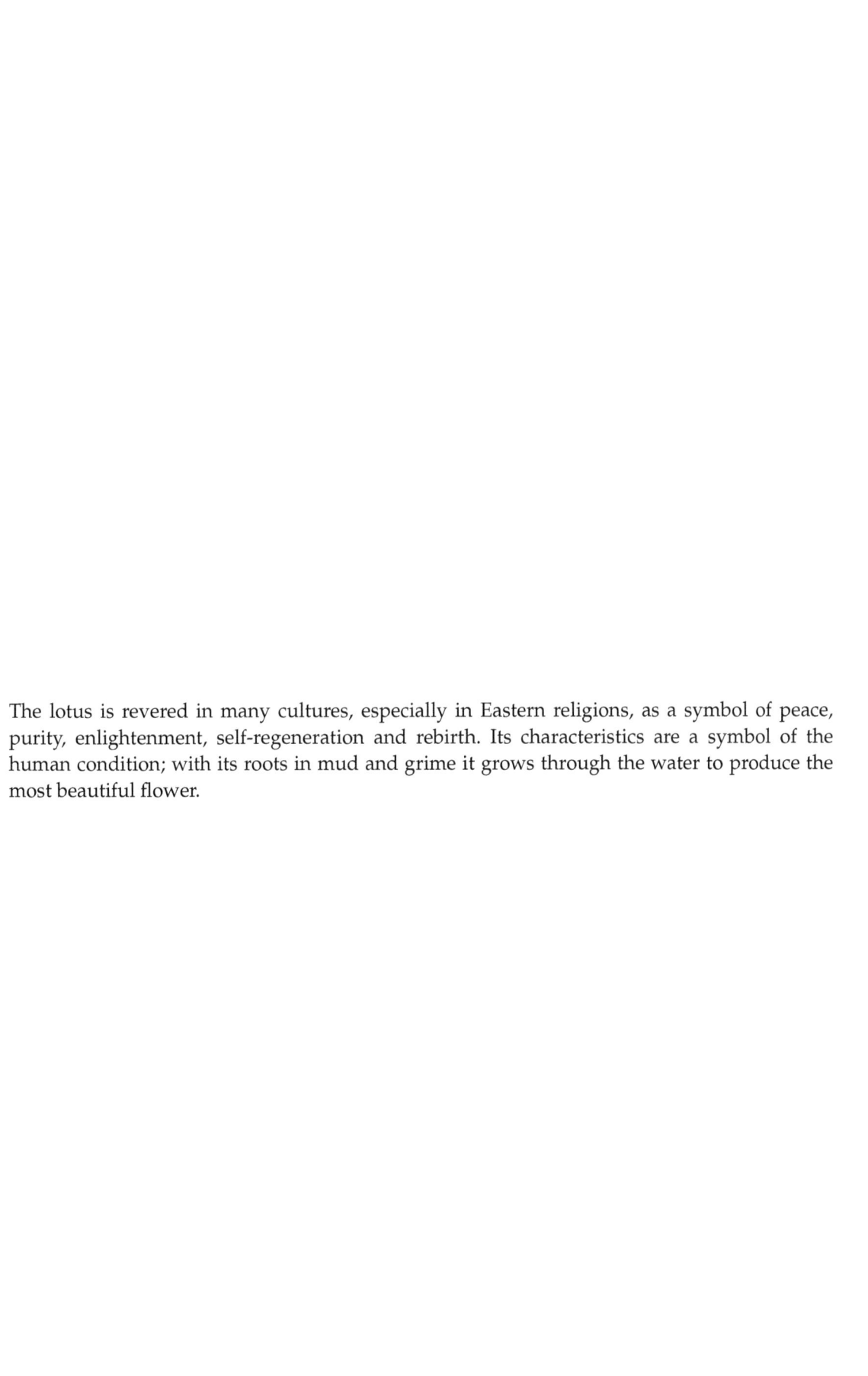

The lotus is revered in many cultures, especially in Eastern religions, as a symbol of peace, purity, enlightenment, self-regeneration and rebirth. Its characteristics are a symbol of the human condition; with its roots in mud and grime it grows through the water to produce the most beautiful flower.

CONTENTS

Introduction	1
The vital person	5
Therapeutic principles and terminology	7
The integrated person	17
The psychology and neurobiology of integration	27
The interpretation of clinical signs	53
Case histories with analysis and interpretation	69
Herbs for integration and harmony	83
Prescribing	93
Tonics and adaptogens	107
The nervous system	139
The cardiovascular system	157
The digestive system	173
The liver	187
The respiratory system	201
The urinary system	213

The female reproductive system	221
The male reproductive system	239
The thyroid	247
The muscular-skeletal system	253
Dermatology	269
References	*283*
Index	*287*

Introduction

> The spirit of emptiness is immortal.
> It is called the Great Mother
> Because it gives birth to Heaven and Earth
>
> It is like a vapour,
> Barely seen but always present
>
> (Lao Tao, *Tao Te Ching*, verse 6)

It might be argued that Western herbal medicine is uncertain of the particular paradigm that it embraces, or perhaps, put another way, it embraces a number of paradigms. In part it follows the reductionist, biomedical approach to health of orthodox medicine, which adopts evidence-based practice. The foundation of this therapeutic approach is in pathophysiology. Pathophysiology provides a structural understanding of the body in terms of the anatomy of the tissues and organs and a functional understanding in terms of underlying physiological processes. This approach lends its self to the understanding and intervention concerned with symptomatic treatment and health management and can be remarkably effective in areas such as surgery and the management of acute illness and symptoms. However, this therapeutic approach does not allow for the understanding of the process by which people become ill and allows little conceptual understanding of people in terms of their functional modalities, which we know as feeling, mind and spirit. This has led to the development of a medical system which does not recognise the emotional nature of man or the importance of the processes of feeling, thinking, intuition and belief. The same can of course be said for the practice of herbal medicine from a biomedical perspective. Illness is conceptualised as an unfortunate circumstance. The differences between a holistic and constitutional approach to treatment and the orthodox biomedical approach at first seem incompatible, but this is largely because of the lack of understanding of the medical interpretation of holism. In fact, the spirit–mind–body axis is understandable and explicable in terms of psycho-physiological processes and principles. It is really a matter of interpretation and adaptation of principle.

In many traditional systems of medicine, illness is seen as a consequence of the breakdown of the integration of the individual, both internally and in their relationship to the world. A holistic view of well-being conceives well-being as engendered by living in accordance with the laws of nature, so that the health of the body, mind and spirit is supported by a fundamental balance and integrity. This holistic perspective has much in common with the ideas of Taoism and other Eastern approaches and is generally understood as originating from the Eastern tradition, but an understanding of a dynamic and integrative approach to health is also part of the Western tradition. The Anglo-Saxons with their concept of the 'Wyrd' had much in common with the traditions of the East. Wyrd in this sense means unfathomable or mysterious and refers to the idea that the individual lives in a web of creation, which is of their own production, and that disease patterns are the consequence of disturbances created by the individual intent and action. The Anglo-Saxon tradition, as well as other early traditions, are poorly recorded, having been predominantly an oral tradition. Contemporary holistic medical systems mark a re-emergence of a different way of looking both at the individual and at the way he relates to the world.

Physiological processes are controlled and regulated by homeostasis involving complex factors, some of which are local to the tissues and organs, whilst others are concerned with the regulation of the physiology in relation to the external environment. This neurobiological homeostatic control is regulated, principally, by the autonomic nervous system (ANS) in conjunction with the central nervous system (CNS). The ANS is largely operated by the older centres of the brain, the limbic system in particular, and forms a large part of what we regard as the subconscious part of the mind. The limbic system is largely concerned with the homeostatic control of physiological processes, such as temperature, appetite, and memory, but also predictability, emotional experience and the expression and coordination of involuntary behaviour, and emotional response.

The sense of self is, however, more concerned with the conscious mind. We are used to making decisions and having a sense of autonomy and free will, which are functions connected with processes structurally located in the higher brain centres and the cerebral cortex in particular. There is a tendency for modern man to experience a dissociation between the conscious and the unconscious and to regard physiology as being unconnected with self. It is usual for a person to identify their self as their verbal self. The verbal self no doubt has some objective assessments, but also includes beliefs as well as confabulations about self. This is the reason why the individual finds it difficult to recognise or understand the non-verbal existential self, or primal self, which determines physiological processes and reactions. As physiological reactions and processes are determined by the primal self, they provide an interpretation of how the primal self is responding. Many people experience a sense of separation, insecurity and disconnection, feeling that they are separated from their sense of self, their heart and their true feelings. This comes as no surprise in consideration of the culture in which they have been raised; a culture that places value on individuality and independence, the transcendence of intellect above feeling, and reliance on external validation.

It is imperative to recognise that physiological function is inseparable from the energy associated with it and the feeling that either created it or accompanies it. A holistic approach involves changing the physiological state and the underlying emotional energy or feeling associated with it and demonstrates holistic resolution. In fact, the physiological pattern can inform the practitioner of the subconscious experience of the patient. Many physiological imbalances resulting in disease conditions in adulthood are related to emotional and psychological disturbance from early childhood experience.

Traditionally herbs are classified into categories based upon their main physiological actions on the tissues and organs, for example, stimulants, relaxants, astringents, sedatives, demulcents, nervines. However, the same herbs can be seen in a different way and as working at a different level. Their actions can be interpreted, labelled and applied differently, to demonstrate how they may bring about a deeper integrating action within the body, connecting the physiological with the unconscious and conscious. This can lead to a change in personal perception and feeling and consequently a change in one's appreciation of the ability to inter-relate in one's life. This is inevitably a qualitative process and individual in approach.

The material in this book provides a qualitative interpretation of herbal actions, based upon and evidenced by clinical practice. This is both the collective experience of herbal medicine practitioners, as recorded in the literature, and the author's own experience over many years of clinical practice. A case history can demonstrate that a particular therapeutic intervention can be effective, but the effects of the medicine are not necessarily reproducible, as the circumstances and context are always pertinent only to the individual being treated. However, it is evidence that a herbal intervention can work in suitable circumstances. It is not claimed that a remedy has an enduring or reproducible therapeutic action, and it is not the intention here to produce standard remedies but rather to explore the therapeutic process and effectiveness in appropriate circumstances. In reality, even in mainstream medicine, where remedies are standardised for symptomatic effect, the effectiveness and clinical outcomes are not necessarily predictable for any particular patient. Quantity is of less importance when prescribing energetically, and the laws of pharmacy less relevant. Lower dosages tend to work more subtly and deeper, they are qualitative rather than quantitative. Energetic actions are more impressionistic and work on the 'feeling' dimension. Feeling is what ultimately determines physiological function. The therapeutic process used is one of active patient engagement, i.e. it is the patient's response to the intervention that determines the therapeutic outcome, rather than the intervention directly determining the outcome. Although the patient may share their story with the practitioner, psychotherapy is not required, this is an organic, holistic process where the psycho-physiological response results in an emotional and behavioural change and hence a change in the context of the problem and the possibility of resolution.

The vital person

> Mastery of the world is achieved
> by letting things take their natural course.
> If you interfere with the way of Nature,
> you can never master the world.
>
> (Tao Te Ching)

The Tao is a system that fundamentally encompasses balance in life. Within reflects what is without. A movement in one direction enhances the movement in the opposite direction. To live within balance is to live in the heart, to be centred and to let go of intellectuality. This requires a 'sense' of trust in a process greater than one's self, i.e. beyond the understanding and control of the ego and a true 'letting go'.

A holistic view of well-being has much in common with the ancient Chinese concepts of Taoism. Within Taoism, well-being is engendered by living in accordance with the laws of nature so that the health of the body, mind and spirit are supported by a fundamental balance and integrity. The person is not sick because of a disease, they are diseased because they are sick. The goal of the physician is to assist the patient in treating illness and to educate them in the ways in which they are hindering themselves. There is a danger that incorrect treatment of disease conditions can hinder the understanding of the real nature of the causative factors. Well-being of the spirit is associated with a lack of desire and concern, which allow for the uninterrupted, spontaneous and harmonious expression of life. Over concern, over work, striving, negative emotional states and negative experience all corrupt this expression and create disharmony.

Holistic medical systems rely on the understanding that the body is dynamic and that an understanding of physiological function requires a knowledge of action as well as of structure. Physiomedicalism used the term vital force to denote the active energy that moves through the body and determines dynamic activity. To understand how the body is working it is necessary to discover what are the pertaining psycho-physiological dynamics and how this relates to the psycho-social integration of the individual.

The American Holistic Health Association (AHHA) promotes holistic health as an approach to creating wellness, which encourages you to

- Balance and integrate your physical, mental, emotional and spiritual aspects
- Establish respectful, cooperative relationships with others and the environment
- Make wellness-orientated lifestyle choices
- Actively participate in your health decisions and healing process

(Walter, 2019)

Therapeutic principles and terminology

The essential factors necessary to consider when evaluating constitutional health.

Illness is always meaningful

Western medical terminology has no aetiological explanatory value or meaningfulness. The manifestation of an illness is a direct expression of the circumstances that created it and, therefore, is a signifier of the underlying process. This is in accordance with the concept of life as a creative interwoven process rather than as cause and effect.

Western medical diagnosis and differential diagnosis

A medical diagnosis can be useful to enable a discrimination to be made of the seriousness of a condition, whether further medical investigation is required, and whether to refer to a medical or other practitioner. However, a specific medical diagnosis is not necessarily required for treatment, as the indications for treatment can be determined from a deconstruction of the case. The ultimate cause of most disharmony is threat. Threat leads to changes in autonomic regulation, endocrine dysfunction and immune reaction (inflammation). It is important to consider that the diagnosis or understanding of the case is the main determinant for the principal considerations in the treatment strategy. For example, a diagnosis of inflammation could lead to treatment with anti-inflammatories, where a deeper analysis may suggest that the inflammation is the consequence of an immunological response to a potential threat and hence lead to a more holistic treatment strategy.

Every emotional response has a behavioural component, an autonomic component, and a hormonal component. The hormonal component includes the release of epinephrine, an adrenal-medullary response that occurs in response to stress and that is controlled by the sympathetic nervous system. The major emotion studied in relation to epinephrine is fear.

(Mezzacappa et al., 1999)

Constitution

The understanding of the dynamics of the physiological patterns and interconnections that underpin the working of the body. The movement of the vital force and the obstructions to its flow.

Functional v organic disorders

Health problems may relate to issues of functional imbalance or compromised organ or tissue integrity, the one being a further development of the other. Generally speaking, pathophysiology is concerned with the resultant tissue or organ abnormality, but not necessarily the functional disturbance that created it, perhaps over a long period of time. Functional disturbance provides an insight into how the body is responding to the situation in which it finds itself, can be assessed from the signs and symptoms, and demonstrates a normal, excess or deficiency pattern. Excess involves an outward movement with or without a pattern of constraint, deficiency involves a withdrawal, with or without a pattern of constraint.

Functional illness is relatively easy to treat, as it is essentially an expression of the person's disharmony and they have a high degree of control over its expression. The patient may be persuaded to change their manifestation for many different reasons, this may include the intervention of the medicine or something about the patient/practitioner relationship. The question is whether our intervention really changes anything or only alters the manifestation of the problem. Organic illness, by its nature, is more deeply embedded, dissociated, and therefore more difficult to treat.

Seriousness of the problem

There is a difference between potential energy and realised energy. The energy status of the individual may be good but not capable of being realised because of the state of the functional organisation, i.e. they are deficient. On the other hand, the apparent energy status may be artificially high and not coherent with the true energy potential, i.e. they are in an excess pattern. For example, someone with significant fatigue may present with apparently good energy but are in fact activated by a stress hormone response that leads to an excess pattern. However, the quality of the energy is different, e.g. one of agitation. Also, the excess pattern is not sustainable and the fatigue becomes apparent when they are not working, e.g. in the evenings and weekends there is considerable fatigue.

It is necessary to assess the depth, extent, and level of the problem, e.g. at the level of the tissue, organ, or organ system.

Deficiency v depletion

The vital function of an individual is a combination of the underlying energy status or energy potential and the degree of activation and interconnection with the world associated with it through neural, neural-endocrine or endocrine control or stimulation. Deficiency indicates that the vital response is inadequate to deal appropriately with the circumstances of the individual. This can be either active or passive in nature or a combination of both. Active deficiency is a consequence of an internalisation of function or withdrawal, as a result of difficulty dealing with the external circumstances or due to poor motivation. Passive deficiency is a consequence of internalisation of function due to a lack of the resources necessary to engender a vital action. Passive deficiency relates to a state of depletion, but depletion can be overcome, at least in the short term, by the initiation of excess stimulation, e.g. an adrenergic or stress hormone activation. In this case the individual may be depleted but not expressing signs of deficiency of activation. In older individuals this may act as a compensatory mechanism and may become apparent in the dramatic reduction in vitality when the response is not essential such as at weekends and when on holiday. Depletion refers to the energy potential of the individual or degree of fatigue, this can be of different levels from easily recoverable tiredness to exhaustion at the tissue and organ level.

The ANS balance/neuroendocrine status

The control and regulation of physiology through the autonomic system and neuroendocrine systems that control the orientation of the body to the psycho-social environment. The neuroendocrine system provides the degree of activation in support of the ANS through the neurotransmitters, e.g. catecholamines, serotonin, melatonin, dopamine. Autonomic regulation will determine the efficiency of the circulation of the blood and fluids and the degree of tissue congestion.

Fundamental energy state or foundation energy

> Inward calm cannot be maintained unless physical strength is constantly and intelligently replenished.
>
> (Buddha)

The fundamental energy state, or foundation energy, is a construct that encompasses the integrated action of the endocrine system, particularly the adrenal glands, together with the other vital organs and the nervous system. It can be conceived as a type of battery status. The fundamental energy state determines the status of activity, well-being and potential of all of the organ systems.

As the Chinese saying goes, 'in the presence of abundant Yin, the Yang is boundless'. A strong energy foundation is critical for the treatment and recovery of all conditions.

Congestion

Excessive accumulation of blood, lymph or interstitial fluid in a tissue or organ. This interferes significantly with efficient functioning, resulting in diminished organ or tissue energy potential, decreasing oxygenation, reducing elimination of toxins and reducing the supply of nutrients. Congestion can relate to mucus congestion or phlegm, where the mucous membranes are hyperaemic and hyper-secretory. Congestion may be caused by local irritation or infection or a consequence of deficiency or depletion factors. Mucous membranes may be affected by irritation, inflammation or infection, all of which create mucus and frequently occur together.

Constraint

Constraint refers to the interruption or impediment to the flow of blood, usually through constriction of the smooth muscle of the arteries. Smooth muscle is in a dynamic state of relaxation and tension with an optimum where there is free flow of blood but with a degree of tonicity. This is largely controlled via the autonomic nervous system. Increased tension impedes blood flow and requires an increase in cardiac output to maintain circulatory efficiency. Many factors, including primarily physiological mechanisms, affect smooth muscle tension, but the main factor is psychological guarding. This is a reflex mechanism to either block the surfacing and expression of emotion or the blocking of perceived external threat and can be seen as a kind of flinch mechanism in response to something perceived as problematic.

Fire

Fire can mean heat and is associated with externalisation of function and movement. A lack of externalisation and movement can result in internal heat. Fire can also mean the externalised assertion of the vital element of self. When it is not externalised, fire may be expressed neurotically through false fire, e.g. patterns of behaviour, such as passive-aggressive, destructive criticism, negative complaining, irritability.

Heat

Heat is related to the concept of fire. Physiologically it can be seen as a precursor to inflammation but is not necessarily measurable by inflammatory markers. It is a combination of inflammatory cytokines, histamine and other inflammatory factors associated with an internalised immune response. Immunological vigilance mirrors autonomic vigilance, i.e. boundaries being invaded but an appropriate response cannot be generated and will relate particularly to autonomic sympathetic deficiency. Heat will seek release and may track through different organ systems creating an inflammatory response and different symptoms dependent upon the organ involved.

Organ activation v organ energy potential

The energy potential of an organ determines the capacity for normal functional activation. If an organ is activated beyond its potential there is a danger of deficiency and depletion of the organ leading to disease processes.

Sympathetic tone

A term which is confusingly used in a number of ways. It can refer to the status of the ANS, i.e. the degree of activation of the sympathetic pathways and hence increased or decreased tone or arousal. It can also refer to the fight or flight response by the adrenal medulla, i.e. a general activation that comes from adrenaline.

Blood quality issues

In addition to the quantitative blood issues, there are qualitative blood issues. These include the anaemias arising from nutrient deficiency and poor blood production and volume. In herbal therapeutics there is the concept of blood deficiency, which relates to the inability of the body to produce blood and circulate it, due to depletion and deficiency factors.

Context

What are the implications in terms of psycho-physiology and psycho-spirituality, i.e. the 'context'? The time line needs to be considered in order to understand the context. A rational interpretation of the context does not always provide an explanation for the primal reactions to psycho-social and psycho-environmental interconnection. The psycho-physiological response is not normally generated from a rational, intellectually considered framework but from the instinctual, primal self. In terms of the emotional and feeling domain, the psycho-physiological response is understandable, even it is not necessarily rational.

Dissociation

A condition where a normal integrated aspect of the person becomes separated and unavailable to the rest of the personality and functions. Usually applies to the separation of the conceptual self, i.e. personality, from unconscious experiences and functions that are unable to be recognised and integrated. This situation may become apparent when there is an incongruence between the professed understanding of the person and the implications of the signs and symptoms.

Embodiment

This is related to dissociation. It involves a change of orientation of the sense of self from an intellectual, head orientation to one which is centred in the body. This fosters a sense of calmness, being grounded and balanced and brings an increased sensorial appreciation of the world and its beauty.

Clinical analysis and interpretation

Clinical analysis needs to be authenticated. Physiology and psychology are a reflection of each other. The clinical signs and symptoms are determined by the psycho-physiological response of the patient to the context of their psycho-social interconnection. The ANS balance provides an understanding of the physiological response, and the tongue provides an understanding of the tissue state. It is important to distinguish what is fact and what is inferred or clinical judgement.

The symptoms are not the disease

Symptoms are a reflection of the physiological disturbance within the tissue and are the body's response to the problem. Symptoms may be:

- Compensatory—enable the body to adapt to the disease condition. Chronicity of adaptation may develop as a consequence and lead to chronic symptomatology.
- Resolving—moving towards a resolution of the disease. May result in acute symptoms emerging from a chronic pattern.
- Degenerative—the disease is progressive and the body is unable to respond adequately.
- Compensatory mechanisms—are generally inefficient and eventually lead to breakdown and degeneration. Degenerative symptoms will emerge when the body no longer has the resources to compensate.

Acute symptoms are eliminative and defensive and demonstrate an effective response to the disease. When chronic symptoms become more acute, it may indicate that the situation is either resolving or degenerating.

Hering's law of cure

Healing is said to occur in the following sequences:

- From the head downward
- In the reverse order from which the disease arrived in the first place and taking about a month for every year the symptoms have been present
- From within, outwards
- The most important organs are healed first

Exogenous and endogenous causative factors

Epigenetics

The concept of the intergenerational transmission of ancestral disease patterns and their legacy has traditionally only existed in alternative medicine, for example, the miasmas of homeopathy. Chinese medicine has traditionally regarded ancestral weakness and deficiency as an important factor in health and disease manifestation. Recent work in epigenetics, looking at epidemiologic and anthropological studies in humans, has demonstrated multigenerational interactions in health expression. An example is the Barker theory, which proposes that the health of an individual is determined by the intergenerational health of the prior 100 years of family members, i.e. the grandparents. It is well known that over or under nutrition of the foetus in-utero can lead to lifelong problems, such as metabolic regulation, diabetes and blood pressure in the offspring. However, these effects can be multigenerational even in the absence of in-utero nutritional stress. The three main factors responsible are said to be nutritional status, the experience of stress and the quality of blood flow to the uterus (Barker, n.d.). Dr Lars Olov Bygren, of the Karolinska Institute Stockholm, conducted a study looking at 100 years of ancestry. It was demonstrated that transgenerational inheritance of epigenetic markers followed ancestral childhood exposure to variable food availability inducing early developmental origins of adult disease (Bygren et al., 2018). Such studies demonstrate the limitations of a view of phenotypic variation based on DNA, clearly the phenotypic variation is due to complex interactions between the environment, behaviour, physiological regulation and adaptation and the genome. The true significance of epigenetics in terms of health has most likely yet to be realised.

Transgenerational transmission of stress

Ghosts in the Nursery: A Psychoanalytic Approach to the Problems of Impaired Infant-Mother is a seminal work looking at the impact of the transgenerational transmission of stress.

> In every nursery there are ghosts. They are the visitors from the unremembered past of the parents, the uninvited guests at the christening. Under all favorable circumstances the unfriendly and unbidden spirits are banished from the nursery and return to their subterranean dwelling place. The baby makes his own imperative claim upon parental love, and in strict analogy with the fairy tales, the bonds of love protect the child and his parents against the intruders, the malevolent ghosts.
>
> (Fraiberg et al., 1975)

Janov (2011) introduced the concept of foetal imprinting, an evolutionary strategy to prepare children to cope with life, which establishes a permanent set point in the child's physiology. The physiological experience of the womb, the birth process and the early years determine many aspects of later mental and physical health.

Conflicts, traumas and tensions experienced by parents and previous generations are in danger of being inflicted upon the offspring and continue to create trauma and conflict in their lives. Many studies have looked at the transgenerational transmission of stress in major conflicts, e.g. Rachel Yehudo has studied the consequences of the experience of the victims of the holocaust on their offspring (Yehuda & Bierer, 2009). The consequences for the treatment intervention are considerable, as it is clear that the verbalisation of the effects of trauma is not always possible, as it may not have been from the direct experience of the patient.

Pathogenic factors

The germ theory of disease is a central concept of Western medicine, and treatment is aimed at the identification and eradication of the pathogen responsible. Many herbs do have direct anti-infective properties, but in herbal therapeutics the emphasis is on treating the terrain and the complex physiological dynamics that underpin the immuno-protective system of the body. The immune-protective system is intrinsically linked to the balance of the ANS and the movement of blood and energy. A situation of deficiency would affect the immune response and vulnerability to pathogenic invasion and also to pernicious environmental influences, i.e. hot, cold, damp, dryness and to allergic sensitivity and to irritants, e.g. smoke, fog, dust, toxins, poisons.

Environmental

Elemental influences

The same factors that control the flow of nature are seen to control human dynamics, and it is normal for the human physiology to respond to the environment appropriately.

> Whoever would study medicine aright must learn of the following subjects. First, he must consider the effect of each of the seasons of the year and the differences between them. Secondly, he must study the warm and the cold winds, both those which are common to every country and those peculiar to a particular locality...'
>
> (Hippocrates)

Folklore and literature often refer to the pernicious effects of adverse elemental forces, but little is mentioned in current accounts of therapeutics. It is certainly the case, in practice, that the person will respond to the elemental forces that relate to their constitutional type. For example, those with a hot, damp constitution are averse to hot and humid weather in the summer and prefer cold or chilly weather. Those with a cold and damp constitution will be attracted to hot, dry weather. In fact, the preference for environmental circumstances give a direct insight into the constitutional type and possibly racial genotype. The question of whether the weather affects health and well-being as a scientific question has mixed results, and studies show uncertain outcomes, with the relationship between the weather and specific infirmities remaining unclear. One study showed a small correlation between the weather and mood (Denissen et al., 2008). Another study looked at patients with chronic pain and found no correlation between depression, as measured by a questionnaire, and the time of year and hours of sunshine (Hardt and Gerbershagen 1999). However, this study did not take into account the length of time that the subjects spent outside. The production of serotonin is directly enhanced by exposure to light and serotonin has an enormous effect on autonomic sympathetic activation and consequently on sense of well-being, vitality, and mood. The effects of the weather may be individual; in one study one-third of girls and one-fifth of boys responded negatively to certain weather conditions, including poor sleep, irritability and low mood (Faust et al., 1974). A German study confirmed that individuals vary in sensitivity with a finding that approximately 30% of Europeans are weather sensitive. Very-low-frequency (VLF) atmospherics called 'sferics' are created by low pressure systems. These are short, weak electromagnetic fields (EMFs) in the 1–100 kHz range that settle down to a common frequency of 10 Hz. Although this is tiny compared with the much higher frequencies emitted by electronic devices, we are very sensitive to these low frequencies, which have proven to have very significant effects on health. (Schienle et al., 1998).

Participants exposed to 10-kHz sferics for only 20 minutes show a large shift in their alpha band (713 Hz), the wave length of meditation and alert receptivity (Tirsch et al., 1994). In our human evolution, the brain may have worked best when tuned in to 10 Hz, the frequency of our alpha cycle—quiet, meditative alertness—and the Schumann resonance, the most common frequency of EM waves that encircle the earth. Changes in sferics may enable the early detection in humans of changes in weather patterns and the capability of early adaptive physiological and instinctual behavioural change. The Schumann VLF fields build up primarily during fair weather, and so it may well be that humans were designed to function at their best when it's sunny and to give in to the impulse to hibernate during stormy weather. Such interaction affects the delicate balance of melatonin and serotonin, the brain hormones that regulate mood, set the circadian rhythm and may be involved (through the pineal gland) with the workings of a number of the major organs. It is the case that complementary medicine practitioners see patients who find certain seasons or the change of seasons challenging.

The therapeutic intervention

1. The prescription of an appropriately formulated herbal medicine for the condition being treated.
2. The identification and control of psychogenic factors in the aetiology and management of the condition and the response of the patient to treatment. Placing the condition in context of the underlying pattern.
3. As far as possible a nourishing and balanced organic wholefood diet where possible. Recommendation of specific changes and improvements.
4. Recommendation of nutritional changes and supplementation.
5. Lifestyle changes where appropriate, such as exercise, specialist exercise, counselling, life enhancing decision making, empowerment.
6. A reduction or control of environmental factors implicated in the condition, such as pollutants, allergens.

The integrated person

> Because one believes in oneself, one doesn't try to convince others. Because one is content with oneself, one doesn't need others' approval. Because one accepts oneself, the whole world accepts him or her.
>
> (Lao Tzu)

> Enlightenment is man's emergence from his self-incurred immaturity. Immaturity is the inability to use one's own understanding without direction from another. This immaturity is self-incurred if its cause is not lack of understanding, but lack of resolve and courage to use it without another's guidance. Dare to know! That is the motto of enlightenment.
>
> (Kant)

The capacity for integration and harmony is dependent upon the ego. The ego serves the purpose of a regulatory system, which acts to interpret, correlate and integrate information from the environment with the status of the internal resources and relate to one's previous experience and the motivations and aspirations of the individual. The ego is best seen as consisting of a number of parts, some conscious and some unconscious, which relate to the different levels of human experience. The subconscious element relates to the biological brain and is predominantly concerned with safety and biological needs, whilst anatomically relating to the limbic brain. The limbic brain contains the processes that assess afferent information, relate this to previous experience and initiate automatic responses through the ANS and endocrine connections. Higher aspects of the ego relate to the ability of reflection and appraisal of ourselves and conscious decision making. The ego is also called the self, which suggests that it is also the element of the person with whom one identifies, i.e. our personal qualities, attributes, values, interests, motivations, and orientations. For some people, this element of the self is limited and limiting, and the true self in reality has much greater potential, i.e. the ego is limited.

The ego and its expression can be severely distorted and may emphasise where there have been problems with recognition, respect and security in personality development. This can lead to overcompensation, which is neurotic in that it can never achieve sufficient value as a replacement emotion to adequately fulfil the sense of inadequacy. Part of the role of the ego is to invest value in one's self. This is normal in a well-adjusted individual but again can become inflated by the need to invest in overcompensatory value.

Egotism is the doctrine that individual self-interest is the appropriate motive and valid end of all conscious action. Egotism manifests itself as excessive rationalisation, denial or narcissism, as well as the inordinate concern for oneself or a tendency to speak or write of oneself boastfully and at great length. Egotism may also be coupled with an inflated sense of one's own importance to the denial of others. This is a character trait describing a person who acts to gain value in an amount greater than that of the values given to others. Egotism is often accomplished by exploiting the altruism, empathy and naivety of others. Egotism differs from both altruism, acting to gain less value than is being received, and egoism, gaining and giving of an equal degree of value. Various forms of 'empirical egoism' can be consistent with egotism, as long as the value of one's own self-benefit is entirely individual.

> What are the benefits of a healthy ego? For many people who are receiving psychotherapy, the task is to strengthen the ego—to develop a sense of individuality, independence, self-esteem, self-respect, personal boundaries, assertiveness, presence, values, separation from parents, conviction of opinions and perspectives, specific tastes and preferences—and freedom from contrary inner psychological forces, which would dominate the ego. When we have these qualities, we have an ego which can be termed well-developed, well-defined, or 'strong'. A well-developed ego is beneficial in many ways.
>
> (Stout et al., 2001)

Key factors for integration and harmony

Feeling loved and lovable. Without love, one feels undeserving and lacking in value. One also feels inferior, and there is therefore a tendency to seek and promote a more desirable false self to help feel worth and value.

Self-belief. This is engendered by being authenticated and having a strong archetype of self-regulation and control. Without self-belief, there is a tendency to be 'rootless' or 'rigid' in mindset and driven by a feeling of the need to break free from dependency. It is essential that one has a developed capacity for strong and good decision making and the capacity to act in one's interests. It is necessary to break links with domineering influences, e.g. parents. Lack of self-belief and control can lead to the development of inner conflicted personalities, which can become problematic. Lack of self-belief and authority engenders a sense of dependency, which in turn results in resentment (Lowen, 1975).

Narcissism. Lack of nurturing in childhood can lead to the continuation of a child-like obsession with self and self-interest. There is preoccupation with one's needs and wants and a lack of capacity to see the need for the benefit of others. In fact, self enhancement is achieved by denying the needs of others at their expense.

Orientation. Tensions that result from unresolved trauma can cause dissociation within the self and create conflicted personalities. Ideally one would have a sense of one's self in one's core, the 'essence'. The educational and instructive processes do, however, often keep the focus of self in the head. This causes a sense of disconnection from one's true self and one's feelings.

In psychotherapy there is a distinction between the true self and false self, proposed by Winnicott.

> Winnicott uses the term 'false self' to describe the defensive organization formed by the infant and child as a result of inadequate mothering or failures in empathy. Experiencing either maternal impingement or emotional withdrawal, the infant is forced to accommodate his own needs to the conscious and unconscious needs of those upon whom he is dependent. Winnicott (1960a) states that the infant's compliance 'is the earliest stage of the false self, and belongs to the mother's inability to sense her infant's needs' (p. 145). Thus, the false self develops as the infant is repeatedly subjected to maternal care that intrudes upon, rejects, or abandons his experience. As a result, the growing child increasingly loses his sense of initiative and spontaneity, as 'there is a growing sense in the individual of futility and despair'.
>
> (Daehnert, 1998)

The developed true self enables a sense of 'aliveness' and vitality, belief in oneself and the capacity that one's actions will make a difference. Residency within a false self requires compliance with an external conceptual reference, and inevitably the compromise to one's true self can engender a deep resentment. One's true self is not a self in any way that can be conceptualised, as to conceptualise it will make it a false self. The true self cannot be known, only experienced as a state of being.

> Prior to all our verbal reflections, at the level of our spontaneous, sensorial engagement with the world around us, we are all animals.
>
> (Abram, 1996, p. 57)

The true self is the feeling self, but it is a self that must be hidden and denied. Since the superficial self represents submission and conformity, the inner or true self is rebellious and angry. This underlying rebellion and anger can never be fully suppressed since it is an expression of the life force in the person, but because of the denial, it cannot be expressed directly. Instead it shows up in the narcissist's acting out. It can become a perverse force. The formation of a perverse primal entity in childhood may be at the heart of antisocial behaviour, self-destructive tendencies and resistance to recovery (Lowen, 1975).

Consciousness can be seen as consisting of a number of different processes, the main two being head conscious and body conscious.

> Many people, especially those who are characterised as intellectuals, have mainly a head consciousness. They think of themselves as being very conscious persons, and they are, but

their consciousness is limited and narrow—limited to their thoughts and images and narrow because they see themselves and the world only in terms of thoughts and images. They communicate their thoughts easily, but they have great difficulty in knowing or expressing what they feel. They are generally unaware of what goes on in their bodies and by the same token, they are unaware of the bodies of those around them. They talk about feelings but neither sense nor act on them. They are only conscious of the idea of the feeling. Of such people it might be said that they don't live life, they think their way through it. They live in their heads.

(Lowen, 1975, p. 317)

This is of course one of the main reasons why talking therapies are not necessarily effective in dealing with emotionally-based problems. Knowing the what, how and why does not resolve the problem. What is necessary is an engagement of body consciousness with the associated emotional or energetic charge. Words can, however, connect with body consciousness is some circumstances, i.e. when they elicit true feelings or emotions.

From the rational point of view of consciousness, the contents of the unconsciousness often seem bizarre and in conflict with the beliefs about one's self. However, the unconscious always feels its truth and this is often uncomfortable with the conscious mind, which has created a framework to suit its beliefs. This situation is often promoted in childhood when adults contradict a child's sense of the truth of their feeling. Feelings are the unconscious communicating with the conscious, and although they are an existential truth, the conscious can decide upon how they are responded to. In reality, where feelings or emotions are deemed by the ego as very threatening, the psychosomatic process does not allow consciousness a choice. The intellect is not allowed to participate in the decision, it is by-passed, and symptoms are induced automatically (Sarno 2010).

There is one neurosis, many manifestations and one cure—feeling.

(Janov, 1996)

Repressed pain divides the self in two, and each side wars with the other. One is the real self, loaded with needs and pain that are submerged; the other is the unreal self that attempts to deal with the outside world by trying to fulfil unmet needs with neurotic habits or behaviours, such as obsessions or addictions. The split of the self is the essence of neurosis, and neurosis can kill.

That pain is the result of needs and feelings that have gone unfulfilled in early life. Those early unmet needs create what I call Primal Pain. Coming close to death at birth or feeling unloved as a child are examples of such Pain. The Pain goes unfelt at the time because the body is not equipped to experience it fully and deal with it. When the Pain is too much, it is repressed and stored away. When enough unresolved Pain has occurred, you lose access to your feelings and become neurotic.

The number one killer in the world today is not cancer or heart disease, it is repression.

(Janov, 1996)

The physical and psychological armouring characteristics of narcissism and other avoidant defence mechanisms can eventually become a prison. Initially created as protective mechanisms, they can become so wired into the brain and personality structures that they require a dramatic, life-altering event to break through them. These 'cosmic two-by-four' events, not only shatter the defence system, but often trigger the early and very dissociated memories that initially caused the individual to build an inflated counter-dependent false self. These wake-up calls shatter the false self and drop the person into the Black Hole, a place where people feel shattered, alone and in despair (Weinhold & Weinhold, 2017).

In Jungian psychology, any unconscious aspect of the personality that is rejected or not identified with by the ego constitutes the 'shadow' or the dark side. In a general sense, and following the Freudian view, the shadow can represent everything of which a person is not fully conscious. The shadow may create a negative projection onto others as moral judgement. The shadow is not necessarily negative, in can contain elements of the self that are essentially more real but not integrated into consciousness.

Winnicott (1960b) could be seen as being unduly optimistic, giving the impression that the removal of the obscuring blanket of the false self would give rise to the spontaneous eruption of the true self. However, the true self will not have developed, and the ego is unlikely to let go of a false self and face an existential crisis. If a true self can be developed, through appropriate experience, the empty grandiosity of the false self may allow the expression of a new sense of autonomous vitality. Miller notes that the deconstruction of the false self in therapy can result in an existential crisis, resulting in psychological breakdown and the person embracing the false belief systems promoted by sects, i.e. becoming less autonomous (Miller 1981a). It could, however, be considered less pathological to identify with the damaged remnants of the self rather than to attempt coherence and identification with the false self at the cost of one's autonomy.

The philosopher Michel Foucault took issue more broadly with the concept of a 'true self' on the anti-essential grounds that the self was a construct—something one had to evolve through a process of subjectification, an *aesthetics* of self-formation, not something simply waiting to be uncovered: 'we have to create ourselves as a work of art' (Foucault, 1983).

> A human being is a part of the whole, called by us universe, a part limited in time and space. He experiences himself, his thoughts and feelings as something separated from the rest, a kind of optical delusion of his consciousness. This delusion is a kind of prison for us, restricting us to our personal desires and to affection for a few persons nearest to us. Our task must be to free ourselves from this prison by widening our circle of compassion to embrace all living creatures and the whole of nature in its beauty.
>
> (Einstein)

The unconscious takes its directions from the conscious, but where this is lacking will take direction from elsewhere or default to previous patterns, if direction is lacking. It is critical therefore that the direction, whether deliberate or otherwise, is helpful and useful. For example, continual self-criticism and negative comment will have a destructive effect on the well-being and integrity of the sense of self. The regulation of the self needs to be under the control of the observing ego. The observing ego is able to maintain a state of perspective and discrimination on the state of the mind, this enables a state of independence of decision making. In fact, it is difficult to imagine that true personal growth is possible without a strongly developed observing ego.

Many problems are maintained out of a mindset of lack of capability or weakness, and the essence of personal growth is the development of personal strengths. Useful strengths include: fortitude, adaptability, flexibility, resilience. These go with the belief system that one doesn't have to be perfect to have a good life, and that all problems do not have to be solved. The resolution of a conflicted self can be resolved by nurturing a strong sense of self. A strong sense of self acknowledges the intrinsic worth of one's self; a strong sense of self affirms one's authority, demonstrated by a capacity to make constructive decisions in one's own best interests. It is important not to be goal directed when undergoing transformative processes. Setting targets that the unconscious may perceive as impossible to achieve or hopelessly at counterpoint to one's self-belief, is a futile process. Change is best seen as a continuous and flexible process of adaptation.

For the unconscious, experience is key; in other words, experience is an existential truth. You cannot persuade the unconscious that something that happened didn't happen, that is a route to denial. You can, however, alter the interpretation of experience, place experience in context and use experience for self-development. The unconscious operates on mindsets or programming, which are the result of past decision making or influence, some of which are positive and useful, and some of which are negative and unhelpful. The observing ego must decide which mindsets are unhelpful. Minds sets can be changed as any habit can. Reprogramming requires an attitude of kindness and firmness, as well as confidence in the outcome and persistence in affirming the change.

In order for toddlers to 'individuate', or become separate individuals, they must learn how to tolerate the loss of their infantile illusion that they are the centre of the world. They must learn how to control their feelings of infantile rage when others set limits for them, or around them. During this painful process, toddlers need not only the understanding support of their mothers, but also the empathic support completed on schedule, or it will continue to cause relationship problems for them later in life. People who do not go through this rage reduction process during their toddler years are likely express rage in their adult relationships, when someone or life circumstances impose limits on their behaviour. As the defences against the need for emotional intimacy become stronger over the course of a person's lifetime, this behaviour can turn into a full-blown narcissistic personality disorder. The massive number of narcissistic adults in the world has become a global problem. As so many people did not experience healthy narcissism and go through the developmental process of ego reduction, they continue to act like entitled, grandiose, euphoric and omnipotent two- and three-year-olds. As adults, their temper tantrums emerge in child abuse, domestic violence, wars and a full range of dominating, revenge-seeking protective behaviours. They feel entitled to more than their share of Earth's resources and even to bankrupt the whole planet (Weinhold, 2007).

So how can we affect the unconscious and our progression? Through the monitoring and control of our intentions and actions. The unconscious responds to what we regard as important, that in which we place our value. Our treasure is where our heart is. The unconscious will respond to what we value, not to what we say we value. Our unconscious will value what we ask it to value and will do so above and beyond physical well-being and safety if we insist upon it. Similarly, the unconscious will take on board those actions with which we engage with deliberate intention, i.e. it is part of the programming of the unconscious. We need to aim for true self-acceptance of our beauty and inherent self-worth. This is not egotistical, in fact, it is the opposite; egotism is the search for external validation of worth, which is unachievable, or at least transient, and demonstrates a lack of the immanence of true value. The egotist searches not only for what they do not have but for what they cannot have because their search is futile. To search for that which you do not have is futile because it is a search based on lack. By definition you are searching for something you do not have and can therefore never achieve it.

Secure attachment and the encouragement of disclosure of emotional states and self-reflection stimulate the development and connectivity of neural networks, which may enable an increased awareness of internal states and emotional regulation. There is a bias towards the right hemisphere of the brain for unconscious processing and affective regulation, and it may be where negative emotion is held. Research suggests that the insula and cingulate cortices are where the interfaces between the cortex and the limbic brain are found; they play a key role in coordinating thought and emotion with bodily experience (Cozolino, 2006).

In the herbal intervention, it is not necessary to be working towards an ultimate goal in the vision that we see as a truly integrated person (if such a thing were possible). The ideal state of a completely integrated person in a spiritual sense is an impossibility for most people, as it involves not only self-mastery of the emotional and mental life and elemental self but an establishment of freedom from the detrimental influences of negative experiences. These experiences need to be excised or the emotional connotation associated with them changed. Complete and absolute forgiveness and acceptance is required. The focus of the self, or identity, is with the higher self to which all must sub-serve, including the ego. The self-interest of the ego mitigates against the ideals of the higher self, except of course where an investment in the higher self results in self exaltation. Spiritual pride is perhaps the most difficult and intransient form of egotism. However, the impediments to self-emancipation can be identified when they arise and considered accordingly. The authentication of the patient, their value and worth, and their capacity to be independent and free decision makers with a 'sense of agency' (the capability of taking effective action) should be inherent in all therapeutic interventions. The presence of a perverse primal entity in the patient can be a major cause of resistance to change and non-compliance and may be a significant problem in the patient–practitioner interaction.

> We become free by transforming ourselves from unaware victims of the past into responsible individuals in the present, who are aware of our past and are thus able to live with it.
> (Miller, 1981b)

> What is unconscious cannot be abolished by proclamation or prohibition. One can, however, develop sensitivity toward recognizing it and begin to experience it consciously, and thus eventually gain control over it. A mother cannot truly respect her child as long as she does not realise what deep shame she causes him with an ironic remark, intended only to cover her own uncertainty. Indeed, she cannot be aware of how deeply humiliated, despised and devalued her child feels, if she herself has never consciously suffered these feelings, and if she tries to fend them off with irony.
> (Miller, 1981b)

> The greatest enemy will hide in the last place you would ever look.
> (Julius Caesar)

The sensitive person

Everyone has a balance between arousal and boredom at which they are most comfortable, and this varies considerably between individuals. The level of arousal that one person might find stimulating and pleasant could quickly overwhelm a more sensitive person and ultimately lead to a shutdown mode, 'transmarginal inhibition'.

The regulation of arousal is subject to assessment of the context, in the light of previous experience, and an assessment of resources. Resources may be physical, e.g. foundational energy and capacity to physically respond but may also be availability of carers and supporters.

Is there a sensitive type who is sensitive on all levels and becomes vigilant because of overwhelming sensory information? It is thought that perhaps 20% of the population are sensitive (Aron, 1999). High sensory processing is a trait in which individuals are predisposed to a more profound depth of environmental and internal stimulus sensitivity, processing and response (Greven et al., 2019). Those who are sensitive typically present with a lowered threshold to external sensory inputs, a susceptibility to the experience of being overwhelmed, and a greater capacity to feel pleasure from positive experiences (Greven et al., 2019).

The sensitive person versus the highly sensitised person (HSP). The sensitised person would have a background of traumatic experience and be demonstrating vigilance, i.e. readiness or expectation of further potential harmful situations. The sensitive person is considered to have impressionable and sensitive sensory processing systems linked to a capacity of depth of feeling. It would be easy to see how a sensitive person could become a sensitised person through the overwhelming experience of sensory load. The sensitive person would naturally have a heightened affective experience, and emotional and sensory arousal is directly linked with heightened conditioning. The awareness of the subtle can lead to a greater capacity for intuitive insight. HSPs who are able to control their sensitivity to overarousal are generally those who have had responsive carers, who have provided good relationships and an environment of security and good resources. This would make the difference between a sensitive person and a sensitive person who has become sensitised. Anxiety and fear promote the short term stress response based on the adrenergic system and the long term stress response based on cortisol, these together with the ANS elicit further arousal and antagonise the situation. Parents who are too protective or too neglectful, both elicit anxiety in their children. Sensitive people are often subject to negative conditioning from comments and criticism, such as you are too sensitive, you worry too much, you always make a big deal of everything, you are too shy etc. This, compounds a feeling of difference, inadequacy and a lack of self-belief.

Many sensitive individuals, if not all individuals, have the ability to sense the interconnection of the web of life and for many it leads to mistrust, fear, alienation and confusion. The educational and socialisation experience of childhood does not prepare us for the use of our innate abilities, and our intuitive and instinctive feelings are often in conflict with what we are told to be true. The development of the intellect creates an abstract world of language and logic, which may alienate the core of the individual and their ability to relate intuitively. Our mission is to learn the language of intuition and insight and how to navigate the interconnectedness of the world. By doing so we become balanced, integrated and connected. Those closest to us, our carers, determine the context in which we live in the fabric of our existence and establish the foundation of our understanding of the world. We take on this context unconsciously, and it forms the basis of our understanding of the world. The majority of this takes place prior to the development of a sense of personal consciousness, ego and self at the age of 3 to 4. This context is concerned with how we feel about the world and ourselves in relation to it.

The herbal intervention may provide a number of resources to help with adaptation to being a sensitive person. The sensitised person requires mechanisms to over-ride their sense of overwhelm. They require acceptance, trust and self-belief and, in particular, firm but adaptive boundaries. Perhaps the most important element is becoming one's self through a process of affirmation. The key is in the development of regulation and adaptation of the limbic brain by the pre-frontal cortex. The triangulation of the individual, their environment and the physiological response is centred on the limbic brain and the amygdala in particular. The individual requires an effective filtering system that allows for the regulation of sensory information. Hypervigilance can mean that the limbic brain is hyper-responsive to all information, rather than deselecting unimportant information through a gating system. Cromwell et al. (2008) emphasise that gating is a physiological process critical for the filtering of information and evaluating repetitive stimuli and is a collaborative system involving the cortex and limbic brain.

Violet flower essence

Violet flower essence is especially attuned to highly evolved and fragile souls, assisting with self-liberation, self-expression and individuation, while retaining the refined and tender qualities of their feminine beauty. In a sense, violet flowers call out, 'come and see me', thereby, balancing a force of receptive beauty with a new found personal will. The Purple Violet flower remedy bridges the virtues and qualities of the violet with the inner foundation of self-worth and courage.

Positive qualities: delicate, highly perceptive sensitivity, elevated spiritual perspective; socially responsive but self-contained.

Patterns of imbalance: profound shyness, cool and aloof, fear of being submerged in groups (Kaminski & Katz, 1994).

The psychology and neurobiology of integration

The organism as a whole is integrated as a dynamic interaction of many different parts and levels, all of which inter-react in a reciprocal manner. A reaction at the tissue level must have a relationship with the state of orientation of the organism at a higher level. The operation and control of the organism can be divided into the following functional divisions:

- Higher centres—consciousness, conscience, intellectual thought, values, pyscho-physiological interactions and processes
- Autonomic processes—psycho-biological or psycho-physiological processes, the CNS/ANS
- Visceral nervous system—nerve plexuses, the enteric nervous system
- Organ systems
- Tissue states and reactions
- Intercellular states

These have largely evolved from psychoanalytical constructs but have become part of the widely accepted way that we regard how we operate and link to our modern understanding of anatomy and physiology.

> Trust your unconscious; it knows more than you do.
>
> (Ericson)

The unconscious or subconscious

The two terms are sometimes used interchangeably, but in psychoanalytical terms unconscious may refer to processes that have been deliberately rendered inaccessible in order to prevent exposure to the conscious. The subconscious is largely concerned with predictability, i.e. to learn from previous experience, and vicariously, in order to predict the likely consequences and outcomes of current circumstances. This has clearly evolved as a successful mechanism for survival. The subconscious is responsible for the interpretation of information from the physiology and senses and for determining the immediacy of action. The subconscious is also responsible for the synthesis and coordination of information received and transmitted through subtle communication, i.e. telepathy, divination, clairvoyance and also for the inter-relationship with the flow of 'life energy'. The subconscious is related to the older areas of the brain and hence to the biological perspective of the relationship between physiology and behaviour, i.e. the limbic system. The subconscious is concerned with the affective domain of feelings and emotion, intuition and instinct.

Deeper levels of the unconscious are concerned with the fundamental needs of life: hunger, thirst, sexual desire, safety and control. The id of the psychoanalysts.

The conscious

The conscious is principally concerned with higher order decision making and is more capable of considering the relativity of importance of a situation and to give contextual understanding. It is able to give direction to behaviour and also provides awareness as a consequence of understanding. The subconscious relies on the conscious for direction, although where this is lacking it will take action by necessity, based upon previous actions. This action is often one that diminishes function, e.g. paralysis, apathy, autism, and is essentially a default mechanism as a consequence of a recognition that the conscious is powerless in the situation. Consciousness is a state of being self-aware, which to some extent also happens within the subconscious. The conscious allows for the consideration of the importance of ethical, humanitarian or personally important issues. There are clearly important issues regarding personal integrity and authority and the ability of the conscious to clearly and unequivocally direct one's life and internal functioning. The ability to have authority and belief in one's own self directedness is a function of early experience. There is a relationship here to the concept of the ego. In the general sense, the ego is the sense of one's self-esteem or self-importance and it is a mediator between the conscious and subconscious. Impairment in the development and maturation of a strong sense of personal authority and esteem can lead to neurotic overcompensation by the need to acquire and demonstrate self-importance.

The super-conscious

The super-conscious is a source of guidance, inspiration and information. It can be seen either as a higher order of the conscious concerned with complex learning, interpretation, creativity associated with cortical functioning or as the 'God within'. The super-conscious communicates with both conscious and the subconscious. The super-conscious needs to be programmed by the conscious, e.g. if you want inspiration you need to concentrate or think deeply on the requirement. Conscience is not the same thing as the super-conscious. Conscience is a learnt process of right and wrong that involves elements of all aspects of mind, whereas the super-conscious is a process of functioning. There is a misconception that the super-conscious can be relied upon as a source of unequivocal truth, in fact, it is a source of personal truth, i.e. it fully understands the values and intentions that are driving you, your true goals and the important contextual issues. Its action is to serve the individual, and it only reflects back that which is put into it.

Autonomic reactions and patterning

- All physiological processes are controlled by the subconscious through the ANS, anatomically, this is largely concerned with the limbic system of the brain.
- The ANS allows for an automatic behavioural response to an environmental stimulus, which is a protective mechanism and serves the satisfaction of the biological needs.
- Autonomic responses have behavioural, physiological and emotional components. The subconscious is the source of the 'affective' domain, i.e. feelings and emotions.
- The subconscious is primarily concerned with memory, to establish from previous experience what is likely to happen in the future, i.e. it is predictive and forms deductive, inductive and intuitive functions. Learning can also be vicarious.
- Autonomic response may be specific responses to precise circumstances or more generalised behavioural or physiological responses.
- Specific autonomic patterning with little connection to the conscious is automatic and outside of conscious control and once established is difficult to habituate, e.g. a phobia.
- The intensity of an autonomic learnt response is in direct proportion to the perception of its importance, relevance or danger, i.e. it is dependent upon specific emotional arousal and general activity. Therefore, an anxious person who is highly aroused will react more rapidly, intensely and learn more easily when anxious autonomic reactions are enhanced. Increased arousal also increases the likelihood of the autonomic nature of response rather than one which is considered, i.e. with cortical intervention. The essential ingredients necessary for patterning to occur are focus, or concentration, and strong emotion.
- The capacity for arousal is also related to inherited differences in neural processing, i.e. up to 20% of the population are 'highly sensitive'. Highly sensitive people are often unusually creative, intuitive, artistic or psychic, often have problems with boundaries and tend to become overwhelmed by excessive sensory input. This is a natural phenomenon and not the same as neurosis, although the sensitive person is more likely to become neurotic.
- Autonomic patterning is enhanced by anxiety, which in turn is increased by the perception of being unable to influence one's circumstances or environment (helplessness and dependency) and the perception of low rank.
- Childhood experience is often poorly related to the conscious, particularly before the age of 3, and therefore is inclined to be relatively hardwired. The capacity to feel loved and for self-belief.
- The autonomic response continues after the potential usefulness of the reaction and in modern society is often problematic, i.e. responses learnt in childhood will persist into adulthood. Often, as a person matures and develops cognitively, they are imprisoned by their historical defence reactions. Complexes are formed by problematical learning and discordance between incompatibilities of feeling and behaviour.

- The defence reaction comprises the following options:
  - Vigilance—arousal and orientation or preparation
  - Flight
  - Fight
  - Tonic immobility or freezing

Each is accompanied by a set of physiological and emotional responses designed to achieve an objective. The autonomic processes assess sensory information and potential response in respect of a wide range of factors, to determine the most beneficial reaction in relationship with the CNS:

- Severity of the perceived danger
- Resources available—energy potential, potential for success
- Previous experience including vicarious learning
- Motivational and control influences from the higher centres

In modern man, autonomic reactions are often subdued, dissociated, or obscured by compensatory behavioural and emotional strategies. The autonomic processes are subject to complex socialisation processes that regulate and harmonise the individual within their social context and allow for the expression of the primal urges in a way which is acceptable and congruent with society. The autonomic system in itself is amoral. The autonomic processes and the subconscious are meant to be controlled by the conscious, not the other way round, i.e. direction should be given by conscious consideration of the options. The conscious has other considerations not necessarily regarded as important by the unconscious, e.g. those of an ethical, philosophical, religious or idealistic nature.

The learning of responses to situations is also learnt vicariously. The observation of others, with whom one can relate, being affected by a situation to which one can relate, will lead to a potentiation of learning, i.e. it prepares one in advance of what may happen in a particular situation. For example, watching a scary film will leave one feeling vulnerable and anticipating danger. There are some preconceived or hardwired behaviour patterns that are passed on from generation to generation. This is the reason why certain phobias are more common, e.g. snakes, spiders etc.

Patterning is also used for establishing bonds. The intense emotions of love and sex, for example, are extreme but relatively short term and serve to establish a strong bond between partners, which is relatively enduring. An extension of this phenomenon is the use of ritual. Ritual is the deliberate act of forming strong bonds to achieve a particular objective. It requires focus and attention and a strong emotional tone. It used for important transitional experiences in life, e.g. baptisms, marriages, deaths, to establish links or commitments.

- Therapeutic intervention may influence autonomic patterning in a number of ways:
  - Decreasing anxiety—and hence arousal by augmenting feelings of security, safety, control and well-being
  - Increasing resources—energising, strengthening, improving self-esteem

- Demonstrating the opposite—e.g. to affirm to the self establishes self-worth
- Forming new patterns
- Creating effective boundaries
- Using biofeedback, affirmation, yoga etc.
• Autonomic reactions are biological processes that serve the corporeal being and may be in opposition to the development and progress of the higher centres of the CNS or the psycho-spiritual self. The learning of novel solutions to situations may herald the breakdown of historical neurotic conditioning.
• The majority of spiritual movements emphasise the development of control or supremacy of the higher self over the lower self and the cultivation of practices that serve this purpose.
• There is a danger in the therapeutic situation of the practitioner providing the safety and security required by the patient, rather than aiding the patient's own development of autonomy and empowerment, i.e. taking control.
• The symptoms and clinical signs are used to assess the orientation of the autonomic process and give a context to understanding the physiological reactions that are taking place. The physiological process is always meaningful in relationship to the processes that created it, i.e. the subconscious.
• Where the clinical signs are not affected, it is likely that the disharmony is beneath the level of the limbic system, i.e. at the tissue level.
• Under certain circumstances there may be disassociation between levels, e.g. the somatisation of emotional pain; the resolution of psychological difficulties but the continuance of physiological states, responses and reactions; the resolution of problematic physiological reactions but without resolving underlying causative processes.

Autonomic regulation and arousal

Orientation	Autonomic nervous system	Behaviour
Control	**Central nervous system**	Psycho-social interface
Constriction		
Regulation		
Activation	**Neuroendocrine system**	
Temporal	Serotonin	Regulation of arousal and activation
	Melatonin	
	Adrenaline	Hyper-function/hypofunction
	Dopamine	
Enduring	**Endocrine system**	
	Thyroxine	Regulation of metabolism
	Growth hormone	Anabolism/catabolism
	Cortisol	
	Sex hormones	
Trophic	Organ potential	Foundation energy
	Tissue state	Energy potential

The neuroendocrine and endocrine systems determine the state of arousal, tone and energy potential, particularly when the organism is not in state of vigilance. If the clinical signs are normal the current state of vital function is determined more by the serotonin and endocrine systems.

Mechanisms of regulation

- ANS—responsive to the interactions between the person and the perceived environment. Gives an idea of the effectiveness of the interconnections of the individual. It links physiology to the unconscious and consequently to the psycho-social environment.
- Passive deficiency—due to depletion factors.
- Active deficiency—due to inhibitory response.
- Excess sympathetic—activation in response to action against perceived threat (fight or flight) or to overcome depletion factors.

Depletion factors refer to the endocrine system, notably adrenal cortical function, but also reproductive hormones, thyroid, growth hormone. Liver and pancreatic functions and the relationship to sugar control is also implicated.

The autonomic nervous system is inter-related with the neuro-hormonal systems: serotonin, melatonin, dopamine, epinephrine. Generally speaking serotonin gives calm wakefulness, melatonin good quality sleep. Melatonin is manufactured in the pineal gland and is partly controlled by light. Serotonin is very influenced by pyscho-social factors, e.g. perceived status and control.

Energetic patterns and regulation

The ANS prepares the body in readiness to deal with the environment in the best way that it can, using previous inherent patterning, predictions based upon past experience and feedback from the senses. This is a logical process and one based upon instinctual processes that judge the importance of a circumstance by the threat to life and the integrity and intensity of the associated emotion or feeling. The intensity of emotional experience determines the strength of an associated connection and the intensity of response.

The autonomic processes are primarily concerned with the safety, security and integrity of the individual. They are driven by the primal urges (sex, hunger, etc.) and do not have any inherent concern with morality. Morality is an intellectual construct driven by ideas of fairness and equality. The autonomic processes also serve to protect the sense of internal congruence or integrity, probably because this is a self-protective and life enhancing facility that has the ability to compartmentalise elements that are incongruent or distressing. That is, it serves to protect the internal environment from external pressures and to harmonise the internal environment.

The autonomic processes are subject to a socialisation process that regulate and harmonise the individual within their social context and allow for the expression of the primal urges in a way that is acceptable and congruent with society. This socialisation process normally becomes inherent within the system, but can be distorted when the individual does not feel an accepted part of the social structure. Autonomic patterns are therefore physiological patterns, which relate intimately and intrinsically with both the unconscious and conscious and behaviour and involve adaptation to the internal or external environment. They are inseparable from the emotional and energetic components that accompany them.

Autonomic nervous system balance

In general, the sympathetic process prepares the body for activity and response, from day to day activities to the extreme reactions required for fight or flight. The parasympathetic process prepares the body for visceral processes, such as digestion. Many organs receive nervous innervation from both processes, in which case the processes are antagonistic, but some only receive innervation from one of the two. Most sympathetic pathways are adrenergic, and most parasympathetic pathways are cholinergic. It is important to emphasise that patterns of ANS functioning are complex and there may be different types of reaction taking place concurrently. The balance of the ANS will determine the physiological processes prevalent at any particular time and is directly related to how the instinctual response of the individual is reacting to the circumstances they are in. The action of the physiological processes is therefore always meaningful. The control of the ANS is through centres in the hypothalamus and limbic system.

The symptoms and signs of autonomic function are not necessarily mirrored in behaviour, although they will clearly influence it. Behaviour is driven by autonomic processes but controlled by the CNS and subject to complex influences. The ANS will favour situations of structure and predictability.

Smooth muscle tone is a major determinant of physiological functioning, as it both directly determines the flow of blood to the tissues and organ systems and also mirrors the energetic response. Smooth muscle is always in a condition of tonus, this allows for a rapid and elaborate physiological response of dilation or constriction. Most smooth muscle tone is determined by sympathetic fibres, with the exception of the heart and lungs. Within the circulation, sympathetic activity constricts the smooth muscle of the blood vessels of the skin (cholinergic) and digestive tract and dilates the smooth muscle of the blood vessels of the skeletal muscles (cholinergic), and there is little parasympathetic control. Heightened constriction of smooth muscle, as demonstrated by a high diastolic tone of the blood pressure, can be the consequence of physiological factors, but can denote constraint. Constraint is an expression of defence either against a perceived invasive problem or as instinctual mechanism to prevent emotional expression, or both.

The sympathetic system has important links with the endocrine system. Noradrenaline release is stimulated throughout the system to maintain metabolic stimulation and to increase activity. Sympathetic stimulation also acts on the adrenal medulla to elicit an adrenaline response when necessary. The sympathetic system also links with the anterior pituitary gland and through stimulation of adrenocorticotropic hormone (ACTH) promotes the release of adrenocorticol hormones, in particular cortisol. Low sympathetic function leads to hypotonia, high sympathetic function leads to hypertonia, and the net metabolic pattern moves from the catabolic to the anabolic.

Deficiency syndromes

Symptoms will suggest a difficulty or reluctance of engagement with the psycho-social environment and are a consequence of either a difficulty of engaging with the external world as a result of previous experience, perceived difficulty or insufficient resources. Deficiency may be active or passive. Active deficiency would suggest a pattern of withdrawal or lack of motivation, and passive deficiency would suggest a reduction in activation in order to preserve resources. The circumstances associated with the pattern will reflect the causative processes. Active deficiency is likely to occur when the individual is demotivated or faced with a task with which they are reluctant to engage. Passive deficiency is likely when there are fatigue factors and during a period of inactivity, e.g. reported energy status may be reasonable when at work but deficient after work, at weekends or on holiday, and is significant to the body endeavouring to retain resources in a situation of depletion.

The person will show physiological signs and symptoms of withdrawal proportional to the degree of sympathetic deficiency and may show the signs and symptoms of congestion and consequent endogenous heat and toxicity conditions. This is caused by a corruption of the vital force, the 'fire energy', and consequent effects upon the immunological function and emotional undertone. The physiological process is one of hypotonia in terms of overall function.

Physical symptoms of sympathetic deficiency through functional disturbance

Symptoms and signs are proportionate in severity to the intensity and depth of the problem and demonstrate a difficulty in interacting with the environment.

- Fatigue, particularly in the mornings
- Muzzy, dull-headed and problems with memory and concentration
- Muscular tension; notably in the shoulders and neck, muscle fatigue; disproportionate to exertion, lack of inclination to exertion
- Shortness of breath
- Tendency to catarrh, sinus problems
- Weak voice
- Digestive disturbance: constipation or loose stools, abdominal distension, wind and bloating, poor appetite or excessive appetite
- Problems of blood sugar regulation, hypoglycaemia, increase or decrease in weight
- Tendency to cold extremities, but this may be counteracted by endogenous heat factors, e.g. hands may be warm or hot but the more distal feet are cold
- Nocturnal heat, aversion to excess heat, heat with exertion
- Lack of libido

- Emotional tone is low mood or depression, overanxious, pessimistic, introverted
- Irritability, impatience or other signs of false fire manifestation

Neurasthenia

- A deeper pattern involving physical exhaustion
- The adrenals, liver and pancreas are implicated at the organic tissue level
- Physical and mental exhaustion not relieved by rest
- Lethargy, pessimism, depression, lack of will power and initiative
- Social avoidance
- Loss of sense of control and purposelessness
- Coldness
- Hypoglycaemia
- Nocturnal heat
- Lower backache, aching knees, musculoskeletal aches and pains
- Tinnitus, dizziness, vertigo
- Frequent micturition with pale urine
- Disturbed sleep
- Loss of libido with tendency for premature ejaculation in men

Clinical signs:
Blood pressure: comparatively low systolic pressure.
Tongue: pale, swollen, wet.

This may be the result of adrenal depletion or exhaustion as a result of overwork, chronic disease, excessive physical activity or excessive sexual activity. A classic example would be post-traumatic stress, where following the cessation of a difficult, prolonged or exhausting process the sympathetic nervous response is deactivated. Sympathetic stimulation is, however, required for promotion of the endocrine system and is essential to initiate recovery. An individual can stay in a post-traumatic state for long periods of time or indefinitely unless a reactivating stimulus intervenes. Mental-emotional factors may precipitate, worsen or complicate the situation. Experience that leads to shock or fear or changes in circumstances where the person is placed in a situation of vulnerability may precipitate. Conversely adrenal deficiency may result in the engendering of negative emotional reactions, i.e. depression, feelings of vulnerability, fearfulness, feeling of instability etc., which may entrap the person and render them unable to participate fully in society or take control of their life. Although the individual is depleted in terms of physical reserves, the internal state is one of tension and irritability. A deficient response may be the precursor to chronic and severe organic deficient conditions, e.g. ME, chronic fatigue, MS, and can be seen as being a continuum of severity.

A high degree of visceral tension, evidenced by signs of smooth muscle constriction, is possibly a good sign as its absence may suggest either profound endocrine depletion or resignation on the part of the patient, i.e. the patient is beyond caring. An increase in visceral tension may emerge when treatment commences and denotes a recovery of active involvement of the system.

Personal benefits of resolution

The resolution of the problem may require the breaking of old ties, unhelpful mindsets and dependencies, and the establishment of a new sense of autonomy, authority and self-direction. The breaking of self-punitive regimes may also be required, e.g. over working, destructive distractions of excessive pleasure seeking, over exercising.

Treatment protocols

Individual organ systems require assessment and appropriate treatment. General treatment is aimed at: strengthening, stabilisation and balancing. Patients will react badly to too much coercion or 'opening up' as fear is a key component. There should be encouragement to explore, take control in small ways by good decision making and motivation through confidence boosting and personal affirmation. Essentially, if the autonomic processes can experience a preferred mode of operation, then it will engage with that rather than continue with a redundant pattern. Many patterns of operation continue to run simply because nothing occurs to change or prevent them. A process of re-patterning. Taking action automatically raises the symptomatic tone and reduces constraint, e.g. decision making, non-directive exercise, non-threatening social interaction, therapy.

Shock

This pattern is the consequence of shock, fear or other extreme physiological reaction to experience. The symptoms show elements of active constriction rather than passivity and involves the parasympathetic system.

– Cold
– Bright white complexion
– Inertia, prostration, lack of energy with weak arms and legs
– Inability to act or make decisions
– Emotionless

Treatment protocols

Treatment can be difficult as there may be a profound reluctance to re-enter the arena of problematic circumstances. Treatment requires the assistance of deep acting and slow tonic actions and the mediation of higher principles, i.e. shock can be an opportunity for reconnection.

Energy depletion deficiency

Sympathetic deficiency from chronic overactivity and old age lead to fundamental energy depletion, related to endocrine depletion, which leads to deficiency symptoms.

- Fatigue
- Anxiety and vulnerability
- Poor cerebral circulation with poor memory and concentration, dizziness or unsteadiness
- Muscular aches and pains
- Hot and cold mixed symptoms
- Visceroptosis and lack of tonicity
- Visceral overactivity—e.g. loose bowels, frequency micturition, SLUD (salivation, lacrimation, urination, digestion)
- Sleep disturbance
- Mood disturbance

This is a passive syndrome consequent upon depletion. Sufferers, who are usually middle-aged or older, may present with anxiety or stress that is not necessarily in accordance with the context of their experience. Treatment is with tonics, rather than sedatives. Young people typically demonstrate signs of active deficiency but where these are absent may suffer from an energy depletion syndrome. The incidence is occurring at an increasingly early age. The clinical signs are variable, dependent upon the circumstances. In extreme cases, for example, in Addison's disease, the vital response is greatly reduced as reflected in low blood pressure. There may be elevated blood pressure as a consequence of increased activation to overcome the deficiency, or the blood pressure may be relatively normal.

Excess syndromes

Symptoms are of hyperactivity and suggest an overactive involvement with life, e.g. type A personality. This pattern is initiated by emergency or difficult situations. Can be an acting out process to avoid inner conflict. In general, the visceral processes are slowed down, e.g. micturition and digestion, and glucose secretion is increased. The physiological situation is essentially one of hypertonia. Can lead to circulatory tension and disease and in the long term degeneration through exhaustion. May be compensatory, i.e. the activation of the adrenergic system to compensate for fundamental energy depletion, this is one definition of false fire.

- Physical symptoms
- Restlessness, agitation, inability to keep still
- High energetic tone
- Irritability
- Assertion
- Feeling hot with aversion to heat
- Insomnia

Clinical signs:
Relatively high systolic blood pressure, fast pulse.

Parasympathetic excess

- Overactive visceral function—irritable bowel, bladder, lungs etc.
- Constriction of smooth muscle
- Restlessness, irritability
- Hyperglycaemia common
- Headache
- SLUD
- Underlying sense of threat or vulnerability
- Internalisation of immunological function and heat
- Mood—anxiety/fear (but not if only in the enteric system)

Hormone deficiency

- Fatigue
- Hot with hot flashes
- Palmer heat
- Mallor flush
- Dryness of skin, hair and membranes
- Fidgety and restless, agitation
- Overactivity of the visceral processes (through over activation of the vagus nerve)
- Palpitation
- Headache
- Overactivity of the digestive processes (constipation, diarrhoea), wind, bloating
- Bronchial constriction
- Mood—agitation and anxiety

The pattern is related to deficiency of reproductive hormones, PMS, the menopause but also other hormone systems. Aggravated by deficiency and depletion syndromes.

Blood deficiency

A common and important problem, which cannot easily be separated from other syndromes. Symptoms include poor cerebral circulation leading to dizziness, dull headedness and poor memory and concentration, fatigue, palpitations, insomnia and diminished menstruation. In the holistic sense it refers more to a process that is greater than anaemia in the conventional sense and includes issues of blood volume, production and movement. Clearly heavy blood loss from any cause, e.g. trauma, excessive menstruation, leads to blood deficiency, but it is also related to more general constitutional states. A fundamentally diminished energy state, particularly as it affects the digestive process, leads to a diminishment in blood supply and movement. Congestion in the digestive membranes reduces effective iron absorption. Poor digestive energy results in the stagnation of blood in the digestive system, and low energy and poor cerebral circulation following meals are significant symptoms of blood deficiency. Blood building is, therefore, a matter of adequate intake and effective absorption of iron, efficient blood production and a harmonisation of blood movement, which is rarely a matter of simple iron deficiency.

Congestion

A number of terms are used for what is essentially the same condition and include stagnation, dampness and perversion. It refers to the lack of mobilisation and therefore pooling of fluids, notably blood, lymph and the interstitial fluid. Congestion is a consequence of a number of factors, including poor vital function (either general or organ-specific), constriction of smooth muscle (i.e. ducts of organs), blood circulation and dynamics, retention of toxins, inflammation, or infection. Emotional tension and negative primal energies are important factors.

Autonomic patterns are in reality complex with intricate synergy of sympathetic and parasympathetic actions together with contributions from the CNS and cerebral cortex, and interactions with the neuroendocrine and endocrine systems. A person may have symptoms of deficiency but at other times an over-riding manifestation of an excess syndrome. For example, a person with deficiency may demonstrate fatigue and deficiency in the mornings, evenings and at weekends but an excess pattern whilst working. This is due to an adrenergic or stress hormone reaction induced to enable them to function and so, although deficient, they will exhibit symptoms of excess. This will manifest in cardiovascular activation, especially a fast pulse rate. The heightened energy profile will be usually be one of agitated action as the principal component is adrenaline rather than normal ANS sympathetic activation, which accompanied by serotonergic activation. This provides a calm and relaxed activation.

Typically, men are relatively sympathetically active when young and become more sympathetically deficient as they age. Women generally are more sympathetically deficient when young and become relatively parasympathetic with age. Typically, men are hot when young and become cold. Women tend to cold when young and become hot. This is caused by changes in the endocrine system. In men, a reduction in testosterone creates a reduction in sympathetic activation whereas in women a reduction in oestrogen causes sympathetic activation through a direct action on the cardiovascular system. In both cases, extreme endocrine depletion can cause parasympathetic deficiency and consequently reciprocal sympathetic excess. Visceral function is affected generally through vagal deficiency.

Energetic patterns—summary

Pattern	Symptoms	Clinical signs
Functional sympathetic deficiency ANS (Active) Low serotonin/dopamine	Peripheral cold. Sweating with exercise or at night. Lassitude. Dull/muzzy head. Heavy/tired muscles. Stiff neck/shoulders—active constriction. Digestive disturbance. Blood sugar dysregulation. Irritability (from internalised fire). Mood: low, introspective. Sense of disorientation, dislocation, lack of control. Symptoms improve with exercise, exertion or concrete activity.	BP: tendency to low systolic blood pressure. Pulse: slow, deep, weak. Tongue: pale, white coating.
Deficiency from energy depletion (Passive) Continuum towards increasing organic depletion Neursathenia Adrenal depletion Addisson's	Fatigue not relieved by rest. Cold but with intolerance to heat/sweating with little exertion. Digestive disturbance; usually excess looseness. Poor appetite. Dizziness/unsteadiness. Pallor. Problems w memory and concentration. Muscular aches and pains. Emptiness in the neck and shoulders. Lower back ache/sciatica. Visceroptosis. Tendency to catabolic disorders. Weak voice. Mood: low. Irritability, impatience. Sense of vulnerability and anxiety.	BP: high or low dependent upon compensatory mechanisms. Pulse: empty/bounding. Tongue: pale. Symptoms of hypo-tonia.

Causative factors	Treatment
Tends to be more common in the young. Poor sense of self-authority and control. Difficulty integrating internal needs/requirements with external demands/context. Includes post-traumatic syndrome. Leads to energy deficiency depletion through dysfunctional regulation and arousal—neurasthenia, a combination of ANS, and endocrine dysfunction. Commonly relates to poor manifestation of 'self'. Disincarnate.	Develop ego strength with tonics, and empowerment. Externalisation of self. Taking action, initiative and control. Expressing one's self. Becoming manifest or incarnate. Exercise. Sympathetic restoratives. Labiatae are specific for facilitating manifestation: Salvia, Rosmarinus, Hyssopus.
More prevalent in the elderly. Age onset. Overwork. Physical and psychological stress. Poor diet. May be post-traumatic or during rest phases. Tonification. Nutrition support.	Tonics, adaptogens and restoratives. Empowerment and stabilisation. Care with compensatory sympathetic drive as treatment can lead to collapse.

(Continued)

Pattern	Symptoms	Clinical signs
Functional parasympathetic excess ANS (Active)	Overactive visceral function: irritable bowel, bladder, lungs etc. Constriction of smooth muscle. Restlessness, irritability. Hyperglycaemia common. Headache. SLUD. Mood: anxiety/fear (but not if only in the enteric system).	BP: increased diastolic. Pulse: increased rate, agitated. Tongue: heat papillae. Hyper-function of visceral tissues, e.g. membranes hyperaemic and irritable. Inflammatory and immune response internalised.
Shock ANS (Active)	Inertia. Cold. Bright white complexion. Possible loss of bowel and bladder control. Lack of emotion.	
Sympathetic excess ANS (Active) Adrenergic	High energy. Impatient, restless. Hypertonia of musculature. Hypotonia/slowing of visceral processes. Mood: elevated, euphoric, hypomania.	BP: comparatively high systolic. Pulse: full. Tongue: red.
Sympathetic excess with parasympathetic activation	Restlessness, agitation, irritability. Hot with heat aversion. Hyperglyacaemia.	BP: high systolic and diastolic. Pulse: full. Tongue: red, swollen.
Blood deficiency (Passive)	Dizziness/dull headed. Poor. Pallor memory/concentration. Fatigue. Insomnia. Dry skin/hair.	BP: depends. Pulse: weak, choppy, fast. Tongue: pale, thin, dry.
Hormone deficiency Sympathetic excess or deficiency	Hot with hot flashes. Palmer heat. Mallor flush. Dryness of skin, hair and membranes. Palpitations. Mood: agitation and anxiety.	BP: high systolic and diastolic. Pulse: fast, irregular. Tongue: red, dry with little coating.

Causative factors	Treatment
Associated with an underlying sense of threat or vulnerability. Internalisation of immunological function and heat.	Tonification, empowerment, reassurance Parasympathetic drainers and relaxants, e.g. Viscum, Leonorus, Chamomilla.
Acute psychological or physiological threat or emergency.	Physical care. Tonics (gentle). Mediation of the higher principles.
'Type A personality'. Externalisation of function, which may be in response to external pressures or represent avoidance of inner conflict or compensation for energy depletion.	Reorientation. Sympathetic drainers.
Mixed pattern with underlying anxiety (active constriction) with compensatory outward activity.	Dependent upon the particular pattern.
Blood loss. Excessive menstruation. Energy deficiency. Emotional strain.	Includes anaemia in the conventional sense but also relates to blood volume, movement and production.
Deficiency of reproductive hormones (and other hormones). Aggravated by deficiency and depletion syndromes.	Hormone tonics. Pituitary regulators. Cooling herbs. Avoid hot/activating herbs.

Causes of heat not related to core temperature change

In these situations the body temperature remains normal, but the sensorial appreciation of heat and cold changes. Fluctuations in hot and cold and reactivity to heat is common in fatigue syndromes.

Syndrome	Factors associated	Symptoms	Treatment
Sympathetic excess Activation of the ANS sympathetic and/or adrenal stress response Note differences between heat and fire	Associated with activation in response to mental-emotional stress, danger and demand.	Heat and dryness. Red tongue with thirst. Red face. Agitation, insomnia. Hyperactivity.	Sympathetic drainers and relaxants.
Hormone deficiency Often refers to sex hormone deficiency but applies also to the rest of the endocrine system	Associated with age depletion factors, such as overwork, and aggravated by emotional stress (which causes the heat to flare upwards) Not inevitable in hormone deficiency.	Red face, hectic cheeks. Dry tissues and tongue not relieved by drinking. Irritability, anxiety, insomnia, restlessness. Tongue red, dry and without coating.	Tonics to the endocrine system. Circulating actions. Resolution of congestion.
Immunological heat/endogenous heat May relate to different ANS patterns, e.g. sympathetic deficiency: cold peripheral circulation, hot interior.	Immunological disturbances possibly associated with anger and emotional stress leading to tension and congestion. Symptoms depend upon the ANS balance and how this is controlling the heat. May be at the organ and tissue level.	A tendency to irritability, bitter taste, thirst. May be associated with dream disturbed sleep or insomnia, headache. Red face and eyes. May be related to dizziness and tinnitus.	Heat transforming and resolving actions. Include cooling, nourishing and aromatic actions. Counselling.

Neurotransmitter systems—summary

There are four principal systems for activating the nervous system:

- Adrenergic system—particularly related to emotional tone
- Dopaminergic system—related to 'reward' in learning and creativity
- Serotonergic system—waking and general arousal
- Cholinergic system—important particularly for memory

These neurotransmitter systems are related to the neuroendocrine hormones.

The neuroendocrine systems coordinate the interconnections between the nervous, endocrine and immune systems.

- HPA Axis—hypothalamic-pituitary-adrenal
- HPT Axis—hypothalamic-pituitary-thyroid
- HPG Axis—hypothalamic-pituitary-gonadal

The hypothalamic-pituitary-adrenal (HPA) regulatory axis controls the secretion of the adrenal cortex, notably cortisol production. The adrenal medulla secretes adrenaline. It regulates the reactions to stress, energy storage and the immune system. Small proteins released by cells called cytokines may be released, triggering inflammation or hormone release. Cytokines may act at several levels of the HPA axis to induce the release of cortisol and epinephrine. Cortisol and epinephrine act to suppress the immune response, thus forming a negative feedback loop.

The hypothalamic-pituitary-gonadal axis is a neuroendocrine system that regulates the reproductive system. The hypothalamus releases gonadotropin-releasing hormone (GnRH) to stimulate the pituitary to release luteinising hormone (LH), which then signals the gonads. This communication pathway ultimately leads to the production of testosterone, oestrogen and progesterone from the gonads.

The hypothalamic-pituitary-thyroid axis is a neuroendocrine system that regulates the metabolism. When the hypothalamus senses low circulating levels of the hormones T3 and T4, it signals to the pituitary, which then signals the thyroid gland to release T3 and T4. T4 is normally converted to the more active T3, but T4 can also be converted to reverse T3 (rT3). rT3 antagonises the T3 receptor, so high levels can be detrimental.

Important interactions

Oestrogen and serotonin, at optimal levels, are inter-related. Oestrogen supports serotonin in several ways: oestrogen increases tryptophan hydroxylase production, the rate-limiting step in serotonin synthesis; activation of the oestrogen receptor (E2β) upregulates the expression of serotonin receptors (5-HT2A). Oestrogen acts as a serotonin reuptake inhibitor and inhibits monoamine oxidase activity, thus preventing the breakdown of serotonin. Consequently, if oestrogen levels decrease, serotonin activity may decrease as well. Low oestrogen levels may result in symptoms associated with low serotonin, e.g. low mood, sleep difficulties, hot flashes, uncontrolled appetite and headaches. Supporting serotonin may counter the effects of decreased oestrogen.

Progesterone and GABA: progesterone's metabolite allopregnanolone acts at the GABA receptor to increase GABA activity, thus promoting calming effects. Low progesterone levels may result in symptoms associated with low GABA, e.g. anxiousness and sleep difficulties. Supporting GABA may counter the effects of decreased progesterone.

Testosterone and dopamine: testosterone improves dopamine levels, which is important for movement, motivation and cognition. Other benefits for balancing include improved libido and lean muscle mass.

Stress hormones—cortisol and the monoamines: cortisol can stimulate monoamine oxidase (MAO) to decrease the production of various neurotransmitters, including serotonin, epinephrine, norepinephrine and dopamine. In addition, MAO can enhance tyrosine hydroxylase

Neurotransmitter	Function

Noradrenaline
  Nervous system
Adrenaline
  Adrenal medulla
Antagonised by adenosine
  Manufactured from tyrosine
	Excitatory: increases heart rate and stroke, blood vessel constriction.
	Arousal, learning, memory and eating. Bronchial dilation.
	Increases oxygen to the brain and muscles.
	Increases glucose.
	Suppresses the immune system.
	Sympathetic activation.
	The flight or fight mechanism.
	Initiates ACTH release for cortisol stimulation in the endocrine stress response system.

Dopamine	Excitatory: involved in voluntary muscle movements, attention, learning, memory, emotional arousal and rewarding sensations involved in learning and creativity.
Serotonin Produced by the brain stem as well as other tissues. Synthesised in the gastrointestinal tract (GIT). 5-hydroxytryptamine 5HTP in the active form from tryptophan by tryptophan hydroxylase B6 and omega 3 fatty acids required	Inhibitory or excitatory: involved in mood, sexual behaviour, pain perception, sleep, eating behaviour, maintaining a normal body temperature and hormonal state. Serotonin. Regulates sleep. Arousal. Relates to social rank. Reduces pain and appetite. Influences mood. Low levels: increase carbohydrate craving. Tryptophan ingestion—red wine, chocolate, peanuts, cheese. Depression. Poor sleep. Sensitivity to pain increases. Antagonistic with epinephrine. Oestrogen decreases B6 which is required for serotonin production.

Deficiency	Excess	Drug actions
Deficient activation. Depression.	Anxiety.	Caffeine: reduces the ability of the brain to produce adenosine, the 'brakes' of the brain and CNS. Doses of 700 mg can contribute to panic attacks (200 mg is two strong cups of coffee; Mountain Dew is 54 mg). Cocaine: affects norepinephrine and serotonin, and prevents the reuptake of dopamine in the synapse and activate the sympathetic nervous system. Amphetamines: increases dopamine and norepinehrine, and to some extent serotonin and activates the sympathetic nervous system. Scopalamine. Ephedra. Sympathetic tonics (Inula, Rosmarinus, Salvia, Rhodiola, Selenius). Adaptogens.
A factor associated with Parkinson's disease: degeneration of neurons in the midbrain that produce dopamine.	One factor associated with schizophrenia-like symptoms, such as hallucinations and perceptual disorders, addiction.	L-dopa: converts into dopamine in the brain Pheneothaizine: reduces dopamine in the brain Amphetamines: increases dopamine and norepinehrine, and to some extent serotonin and activates the sympathetic nervous system.
Anxiety, mood disorders, insomnia, hyperacusis, photophobia. One factor associated with obsessive-compulsive disorder and depression. Contributes to muscular weakness and stiffness.	Agitation, confusion.	LSD: impairs the reuptake of serotonin, making more serotonin available. Prozac: Prevents the reuptake of serotonin, making more serotonin available MDMA (ecstasy): destroys serotonin nerve cells in animals with moderate and large doses. Oestrogen. Cortisol. Panax and other tonics. Hypericum.

(Continued)

Neurotransmitter	Function
Melatonin Produced from serotonin during darkness by the pineal gland and is antagonistic to serotonin.	Powerful antioxidant that protects nuclear and mitochondrial DNA. Immunoregulator for the immune system. Aids sleep. Influences biological cycles, e.g. behaviour, reproduction. Learning and memory. Increases dreaming
Acetylcholine	Excitatory: it produces muscle contractions and is found in the motor neurons; in the hippocampus, it is involved in memory formation, learning and general intellectual function.
GABA (gamma aminobutyric acid)	Calming. Sleep. Sensory integration. Speech and language. Information processing. Inhibitory: communicates messages to other neurons, helping to balance and offset excitatory messages. It is also involved in allergies.
Neuropeptides Endorphins Enkephalins Dynorphins Endorphins Opoid polypeptide, produced by the pituitary gland and the hypothalamus, produces well-being and euphoria during strenuous exercise, excitement and orgasm There is significant interaction with the endocrine system.	Inhibitory: regulates pain perception and involved in sexuality, pregnancy, labour and positive emotions associated with aerobic exercise—the brain's natural opiates.

Deficiency	Excess	Drug actions
Paralysis: a factor associated with Alzheimer's disease: levels of acetylcholine are severely reduced associated with memory impairment.	Violent muscular contractions.	Nicotine: increases the release of acetycholine. Curare: blocks the receptor sites of acetycholine. Botulin: poisons found in improperly canned food, blocks the release of acetylcholine resulting in paralysis of the muscles. Nerve gas: continual release of acetylcholine. Scopolamine: blocks ACh receptors and impairs learning and even at low doses causes drowsiness, amnesia and confusion.
Anxiety.		Diazepam. GHB. Alcohol. Tilia.
Body experiences pain.		

(Continued)

Neurotransmitter	Function
Substance P	Enhances pain perception Counters the effects of certain nerve-damaging chemicals, and may be useful for prevention or treatment of nerve degeneration.
Glutamate	Excitatory: critical for learning and the formation of memories. It is used by interneurons. Movement and motor control.
Oxytocin	Social bonding. Sexual reproduction. Childbirth and bonding with the child after birth.

to cause an increase the same neurotransmitters, including GABA, if needed. Furthermore, an upregulated immune system can be dampened by increased cortisol.

Actions of cortisol

- Fear leads to the stagnation of growth due to the emphasis of the body towards vigilance against potential threats rather than exploration of its potential.
- Stress hormones shift the emphasis of cortical arousal away from the pre-frontal cortex to the hind brain, i.e. to rely upon rapid autonomic reactions rather than slower consider responses.
- Cortisol can increase or decrease serotonin potential, i.e. in normal situations it increases but in situations of hypercortisolaemia, chronic depression or chronic generalised anxiety syndrome it has little effect, presumably because serotonin production has reached its limit or is compromised.
- Cortisol induced increased serotonin uptake in the normal, control group but not in the GAD or depressive groups, presumably because serotonin transport had reached its limit due to chronically elevated cortisol levels.

(Tafet et al., 2001)

Catecholamines (dopamine, norepinephrine and epinephrine)

'Turn on' our heart and muscles and 'turn off' the stomach to prepare for fight or flight responses during stress, similar opposing actions in the brain may turn on the amygdala and turn off the pre-frontal cortex (higher cognitive centre), allowing posterior cortical and subcortical structures to control behaviour. The amygdala is a phylogenetically older structure in the medial temporal lobe, long known to be essential for the expression of emotion and the formation of associations between stimuli and emotions. In contrast, the pre-frontal cortex expands greatly in primates and permits working memory to guide our behaviour, inhibiting inappropriate responses or distractions and allowing us to plan and organise effectively. High levels of catecholamines exert opposite actions on these brain regions.

Deficiency	Excess	Drug actions
	Anxiety. Hyperactivity. Impulsivity.	Reciprocal with GABA.

- The flight or fight mechanism
- Increases oxygen to the brain and muscles
- Increases heart rate and stroke volume
- Increases glucose
- Suppresses the immune system
- Initiates ACTH release for cortisol stimulation in the endocrine stress response system

Palmer, McCown and Kerby (1997) and Palmer, McCown and Thornburgh (1998) demonstrated that childhood environments high in parental care give improved serotonin levels and social ranking of children. This study looked at the relationship between social rank and serotonin levels in primates and found that the higher the social rank, the higher the serotonin levels. Serotonin appears to provide for an increased range of behavioural movement and hence access to resources. Primates at the lower end of the social rank were of two groups, one which was predominantly passive and acquiescent and the other which made aggressive assertions into the social group when the occasion presented itself. Some primates exhibited an increase in social rank when given selective serotonin reuptake inhibitors (SSRIs), but this has not been apparent in humans. In humans, although serotonin might be the biochemical mediator most influenced by social rank, a host of factors, including numerous neurotransmitters, reproductive hormones and stress hormones are all affected and related to factors of significant cognitive complexity. It is quite possible to be highly self-directed and fairly independent of others, but this only works for a high ranking individual, a low ranking individual might find it problematical with work, social pressures and relationships. The authors demonstrate that childhood environments high in parental nurturance produce individuals predisposed to high-status functioning as adults (e.g., they are highly sociable, responsible, self-controlled and low in impulsivity). Conversely, childhood environments low in parental nurturance and high in family discord produce individuals predisposed to low-status functioning as adults (e.g., they have low levels of sociality, responsibility, self-control and high levels of impulsivity) and have relatively low serotonin levels.

The interpretation of clinical signs

The clinical signs provide insight into the psycho-physiological response and their analysis can provide essential information on the level of response. For example, the blood pressure is related to the balance of the ANS and provides an interpretation of the psycho-physiological response, in terms of the limbic brain. The tongue is reflective of the condition of the tissues and organs. The tongue pattern and blood pressure dynamics should demonstrate a relationship with each other, but they may become incongruent. This often happens with age, as the capacity of the individual to master their psycho-social situation develops with experience and they develop a sophisticated and capable persona, which is incongruent with their deeper sense of self. This is a process of dissociation; a compartmentalisation that enables tolerance of psychological dissonance. This can also happen where there is significant unresolved trauma. An example is the case of a man with psoriasis who said that he acquired the condition at the age of ten, approximately three weeks after witnessing the drowning of his younger brother in a river close to their home. He provided a rational and clear explanation of his understanding of the situation, but with no sign of any emotional concern or connection. His blood pressure was 110/60, which shows no disharmony, in fact, an unusual lack of disharmony, but his tongue was swollen with a considerable degree of inflammatory heat. The rationale is that the emotional disharmony, e.g. grief and guilt, which underlay his condition, was not experienced at the level of consciousness or the limbic brain but was somatised at the organ and tissue level. He therefore had no experience of the emotions that created the condition.

The assessment of the clinical signs from the medical point of view is largely to determine pathological change, and mild to moderate changes are often regarded as idiosyncratic variations. From the herbal therapeutic perspective, the mild to moderate changes are those that reflect changes in functional balance and are the most important to the analysis of the constitution. The clinical signs, therefore, are very significant to assessing the depth and consequence of the therapeutic intervention. Generally speaking, if the clinical signs don't change with the treatment intervention then it is unlikely that true change has been achieved. Conversely, if the clinical signs are relatively normal and hence don't change much with treatment intervention, it is less likely that the patient will experience an improvement in their well-being.

Blood pressure

Opinions vary on what constitutes a normal blood pressure, but there is some agreement that normality is a systolic reading of below 145 and a diastolic reading of below 90. In reality, the average blood pressure is probably considerably above that which is the ideal and this influences the view of what is normal. Blood pressure is considered to increase with age but this is not inevitable and is the consequence of constitutional change or disease. It is certainly the case that for many individuals their blood pressure does not change significantly throughout their lives. The assessment of blood pressure in Western medicine is largely concerned with determining the onset and progress of cardiovascular disease and the taking of preventative treatment, although this view is now changing and the relationship of blood pressure to cardiovascular disease is not necessarily treated as causative.

Observation from practice suggests that ideal blood pressure readings are perhaps:

- Men: 120/70
- Women: 110/60

These are the measurements that seem to pertain in those who report good health and well-being and are the readings that develop when patients normalise when being treated constitutionally. There is however a wide range of variability between individuals. It is certainly the case that blood pressure is understandable by interpretation of the context in which it is occurring, and it can vary significantly during the same day dependent upon the pertaining circumstances.

Probably of greater significance is the pulse pressure (Priest & Priest, 1983). This is the difference between the systolic and diastolic, which gives an indication of cardiac output in relation to the resistance of smooth muscle tension. This gives a better indication of the efficiency of the arterial circulation and the relationship to the ANS. Priest suggests the ratio of the pulse pressure to the systolic and diastolic should be: 3:2:1. Systolic: diastolic: pulse pressure, e.g. 120:80:40 (Priest & Priest, 1983).

However, in practice, a pulse pressure of 50 would seem to be ideal. In terms of the experience of the patient, a normal pulse pressure means that the experience of the patient is one of normality and reasonable energy output, despite what other factors pertain, e.g. a person can be significantly depleted, but in a situation where they need and are able to provide a good cardiovascular output, they are able to function relatively normally, at least for a short period of time. If the pulse pressure is elevated it could indicate that the patient is needing to exert additional cardiovascular output to respond to adverse circumstances, overcome significant depletion factors or cardiovascular disease.

Pulse pressure	Interpretation	Action
> 60	Pathological excess.	Consider pathological causes.
60	Excess.	Tonification. Relaxation. Reassurance.
50	Normal.	
40	Deficient.	Tonification. Activation. Reassurance.
< 40	Pathological deficiency.	Consider pathological causes.

Priest and Priest also mention the concept of the cardiovascular index (CVI), which is a measurement of systolic + diastolic x pulse. This provides for an index of the relationship between the systolic, the diastolic and pulse. They suggest a normal range is between 12,000–14,000; with measurements below 12,000 as being asthenic, depressive or wasting; measurements above 14,000 as being representative of circulatory tension; and measurements above 20,000 as indicative of cardio-renal-vascular pathologies. Interpretation must be in context but can be very useful, i.e. output, arterial resistance, and the heart rate. It is possible for someone to have a low pulse pressure and a relatively high CVI. A situation where the individual is disconnected from their psycho-social environment can be demonstrated by a relatively low systolic blood pressure, but with a high net output as a consequence of a rapid pulse, perhaps due to a stress hormone response.

CVI	
> 25,000	Danger of cerebral haemorrhage.
> 20,000	Cardio-renal-vascular pathologies.
14,000–20,000	Degrees of circulatory tension.
12,000–14,000	Normal.
< 12,000	Asthenic syndromes, wasting pathologies, chronic depressive states.

(Priest & Priest, 1983)

Case history: CVI

A 65 year old man had a blood pressure of 160/70 and a pulse of 50. He was under pressure from his GP to start treatment for hypertension. However, when his blood pressure is considered in relation to his pulse, his CVI works out at 11,500, which is on the lower end of normal. His elevated pulse pressure can therefore be seen as a compensation for a low pulse, and to symptomatically lower this with medication is not only ill-advised, it is potentially harmful.

Pathophysiological factors for increased pulse pressure:

- Aortic incompetence, arteriosclerosis, severe anaemia, bradycardia, hyperkinetic circulation (e.g. hyperthyroid, hypercapnia, AV fistula)

Pathophysiological factors for decreased pulse pressure:

- Ischaemic heart disease (reduced myocardial contractibility), hypovolaemia (blood loss, dehydration), relative hypovolaemia from poor vascular tone (e.g. septicaemic shock)
(Llewelyn et al., 2006)

Systolic blood pressure

The systolic is the upper reading of the blood pressure measurement and is the measurement of the maximum pressure exerted in the artery following ventricular systole. This is a measure of cardiac output in response to physiological demand, e.g. exercise, excitement, anxiety or to overcome circulatory impediment. Short term increases are largely the result of sympathetic nerve action and norepinephrine, longer term changes are more likely to be due to changes in peripheral circulation. In general, increased systolic blood pressure is an indication of an externally orientated physiological pattern, an outward movement of energy and externalised pattern of behaviour.

Cardiovascular disease also causes an increase in systolic output, necessary to maintain circulation against a situation of deteriorating arterial tissue state. However, in severe cardiovascular disease the systolic output may fall due to constitutional weakness and poor arterial tone. Depletion factors may increase the systolic blood pressure, which would be compensatory to overcome reduced vitality or depletion factors. If severe, this may lead to a reduced systolic pressure where there is insufficient vitality to raise the pressure in compensation. For example, in Addison's disease the vital signs, including blood pressure, fall considerably.

Pathophysiological causes of hypertension:

- Obstructive causes (e.g. coarctation of the aorta, arterial stenosis), primary hyperaldosteronism, Cushing's syndrome, acromegaly, drug-induced

Pathophysiological causes of hypotension:

- Myocardial stenosis or regurgitation, hypovolaemia (blood loss, dehydration), Addison's disease/adrenal failure, relative hypovolaemia from poor vascular tone (e.g. septicaemic shock)
(Llewelyn et al., 2006)

Diastolic blood pressure

The diastolic is the lower reading and is the measurement of the pressure in the artery during ventricular diastole; this pressure is largely determined by the degree of contraction of the smooth muscle of the artery. Smooth muscle has a normal state of tonicity and the diastolic will reflect hyper or hypotonic states of smooth muscle contracture. High diastolic blood pressure is caused by a number of factors, the most significant being:

- Vasoconstriction induced by stress and tension
- Vasoconstriction induced by hormone deficiency, e.g. certain stages of the menstrual cycle, menopause, endocrine deficiency syndromes
- Reflex irritation from immunological processes, toxic reactions concerned in food intolerance, allergy, and autoimmune conditions

Stress and tension

A raised diastolic blood pressure may suggest a pattern of constraint due to psycho-physiological guarding, which induces visceral constriction as an autonomic 'flinch' mechanism, a protective reaction to perceived danger. The perceived danger may be the consequence of particularly sensitive or undeveloped emotional and sensory boundaries, often in relation to a sense of vulnerability and lack of personal authority. Constraint may also be an unconsciously mediated autonomic action to block the surfacing of feelings and emotions that are painful or problematic to address or difficult to integrate into the conscious mind and processes (i.e. invokes cognitive dissonance). This is connected to a process of dissociation, where the unconscious mind with its problematical feelings and emotional content is separated from the conscious mind.

The relationship of blood pressure changes to the external environment is controlled by autonomic processes in the limbic system. Disharmony that is not at the level of the limbic system will not register in measurements of blood pressure. In this case, dissociation will not elicit constraint, and constraint may emerge as dissociation dissipated through the therapeutic intervention. Dissociation may result in the somatisation of emotional issues, i.e. the embedding of problems into the tissue and organ level and hence further away from consciousness.

Case history: urticaria

A 42-year-old woman presented with chronic urticaria. She worked in a stressful office environment. She also suffered from frequent headaches, muzzy head and sinus problems.

Clinical signs:
Blood pressure: 120/80. Pulse: 70.
Pulse pressure: 40. CVI: 14,000.
Tongue: pale with superficial heat.

Following three years of constitutional treatment her clinical signs were:
Blood pressure: 130/80.
Pulse: 65.
Tongue: pink with no heat.
This provides a pulse pressure of 50 and a CVI of 13,650.

Although her circumstances had not changed, she no longer felt stressed and she felt much more relaxed and in control. She no longer suffered from headaches and tension and her energy significantly improved. The pulse pressure reflects this change; from a position of deficiency to one of slight excess. The externalisation of function was significant to the clearing of the endogenous heat pattern apparent in her tongue.

Hormone deficiency

The cardiovascular system, along with all other tissues, have intracellular hormone receptors for steroidal hormones (androgens, glucocorticoids, progestins, vitamin D, etc.). Steroidal effects may be genomic, slow and long lasting affecting tissue states, or non-genomic, having rapid but short acting effects primarily affecting functionality. Steroid hormone genomic and non-genomic effects may occur simultaneously and may act at different levels, revealing the high complexity of steroid hormone regulation of cell function (Tostes et al. 2013). Oestrogen in particular has been widely studied and exerts actions on the endothelium, as well as smooth muscle contractibility.

Tostes and colleagues (2013) report:

> A very interesting observation is that the vascular cells are capable of expressing aromatase, the key enzyme in the estrogen synthesis pathway, suggesting that the vascular system is capable of local estrogen biosynthesis in vivo, which may lead to activation of ER and downstream activation of target genes (13). Locally produced estrogen may therefore act in an endocrine, paracrine and autocrine manner on vascular and non-vascular cells.

Postmenopausal changes in oestrogen levels have complex implications for cardiovascular health, which include an increase in arterial muscular contractibility and an increase in diastolic blood pressure. An increase in smooth muscle constriction is a common finding in postmenopausal women and may relate to the onset of hypertension. This is a situation often compounded by stress factors associated with important personal changes in relation to their psycho-social interconnection.

Fluctuations in hormone levels are a likely explanation for the changes often observed in blood pressure readings throughout the menstrual cycle. In the pre-menstrual stage the diastolic blood pressure often increases due to drop in hormone levels and is probably associated with pre-menstrual tension and uterine cramping. This is often associated with a fall in the systolic blood pressure, as the blood tends to pool in the pelvis.

Immunological response

Immunological sensitivity can be involved in cardiovascular changes. An immune response involves the release of histamine and other pro-inflammatory substances, which in turn initiate a stress hormone response. Spikes of stress hormone release create an increase in blood pressure and pulse. Cortisol is the major regulator of inflammation. The more histamine that is released, the more cortisol it takes to control the inflammatory response and the harder the adrenals have to work to produce more cortisol. Chronic allergy is therefore likely to lead to cortisol deprivation or adrenal fatigue (Wilson, 2009). Adrenal fatigue leads to a deficiency state, which compounds the problem. Conversely, sensitivity has a relationship to a deficiency pattern and fatigue. A deficiency pattern leads to an increase in visceral function and consequentially a likelihood of increased immune-mediated response to potential irritants and allergens.

Dr Coca's Pulse Test was developed in the 1930s. A raise in pulse rate follows the ingestion of foods that initiate an immunological response. This is a crude instrument, but when combined with a food diary can provide very helpful information.

The pulse

The pulse is a significant indicator of cardiovascular fitness. Cardiovascular fitness will lower both the blood pressure and pulse. The other main determinant of the pulse is the metabolic rate, and this is determined largely by thyroid activity. A slow pulse can therefore be an indicator of low thyroid function and can be apparent at subclinical levels. This may suggest a secondary hypothyroid function related to adrenal fatigue. In a situation of depletion, the body may use a strategy of reducing thyroid activity in order to reduce the metabolism and conserve resources.

Normal rate is between 60–80 beats per minute.

- Men generally have a slower rate than women
- It increases with exercise, anxiety and excitement
- Exercise increases cardiovascular efficiency and lowers the pulse
- A slow pulse may indicate lowered vitality/energy/endocrine function
- The vagal nerve slows the pulse
- The main factor for sustained pulse rate is the metabolic rate, which in turn is determined largely by thyroid function

Bradycardia: < 60 beats per minute
Possible causes:
Myxoedema. Heart block. Ischaemic heart disease. Hypothermia. Drugs, e.g. beta-blockers

Tachycardia: > 120 beats per minute
Possible causes:
Fever. Shock, e.g. blood loss. Hypoxia. Heart failure. Pulmonary embolism. Thyrotoxicosis. Anaemia. Pregnancy. Drugs.

There are some pulse patterns that are characteristic of pathophysiological conditions and have a defined quality. However, pulse diagnosis is a Chinese medicine technique that is used to determine functional regulation of Qi and blood, organ and tissue states, and disease syndromes. In its full form it is a highly complex and sophisticated technique, which is only explicable in terms of Chinese medicine concepts, requiring many years of practice. The technique probably depends upon subjective observation and interpretation, as well as objective assessment. Some of the main patterns of pulse diagnosis may be interpretable into a useful form for use in Western herbal medicine, however, the analysis of blood pressure and pulse readings provides some of the same information. In reality, how the pulse feels is a direct correspondence to the causative factors.

Factors affecting the pulse

Season	Spring: slightly wiry.
	Summer: soft, round, slightly slippery and superficial.
	Autumn: soft, light and superficial.
	Winter: deep and relatively hard.
	These are reflective of the vital response to the environment.
Gender	Relatively stronger in men than women.
Age	Often weakens in old age but can become full and wiry due to cardiovascular problems.
Body build	Should be naturally stronger, larger, and more robust in larger people and weaker, smaller and shorter in smaller, more frail people.
Menstruation	Usually slightly slippery before menstruation, becoming relatively weaker and slower with menstruation.
Pregnancy	Slippery and becoming more so as pregnancy advances.

Depth of the pulse

In Chinese medicine, the pulse is examined by applying light pressure, medium pressure and deep pressure to determine at what level the pulse is strongest. It is normal to feel the pulse with smoothness and even strength throughout the three levels.

Pulse characteristics

Some pulse characteristics can be objectively assessed and interpreted, e.g. a fast pulse can be diagnosed by checking for pyrexia, anaemia or physical or emotional context. In other cases, an observation and interpretation may be subjective. For example, a 'mutable' pulse is one where it feels uncertain or wavering, this may be interpreted as someone who is uncertain about what action to take or is an individual who has a characteristic of a changeable personality.

Some classical Chinese pulse patterns

	Characteristic	Chinese meaning	Western interpretation
Floating	Superficial. Can only be felt on the surface. Normal in underweight persons and in summer heat conditions.	Yang response to pathogenic invasion. Yin deficiency.	Fever. Extreme energy depletion.
Deep	Can only be felt in the middle and deep position. Deep-full or deep-weak.	Pathogenic factor in the interior. Yang deficiency.	Fatigue. This feature can be detected even in those with a relatively high blood pressure.
Slow	Slow beat.	Cold pattern. Cold phlegm. Damp cold.	Endocrine depletion. Fatigue. Cold.
Rapid	Fast beat.	Heat. e.g. Yin deficiency Full or empty heat and the organ level involved.	Fatigue, anaemia, hormone deficiency, emotional upset, anxiety, ingested substances, e.g. alcohol. Heat.
Empty	Soft, distending to the superficial level, has no strength and disappears with light pressure.	Qi deficiency. Blood deficiency. Summer heat.	Fatigue. Blood deficiency.
Full	Full, hard and long on all levels. Has a springy quality.	Heart, stomach or liver fire. Full cold. Stagnation. Phlegm.	High sympathetic output. Could be associated with fatigue and congestion.
Slippery	Smooth flow and slides under the finger. Feels like pearls rolling in a basin or a fish swimming.	Phlegm. Dampness. Blood stasis. Pregnancy.	Hypotonic smooth muscle tension, i.e. low diastolic blood pressure.
Choppy	Rough, ragged and short without a wave motion.	Blood deficiency. Essence deficiency. Body fluid deficiency Blood stasis.	Feels chaotic. Usually relatively high systolic and diastolic blood pressure.
Wiry			Hypertonic smooth muscle tension. High diastolic blood pressure.

(Maciocia 2004)

Differences between right and left pulses

A difference of 10 mg blood pressure, between the right and left pulses, is considered to be normal. However, differences in blood pressure may be due to factors of the pulse character and detectability. It is common for the pulse on the dominant arm to appear stronger and louder, and is due to the pulse being more superficial, and as a consequence it is easier to detect and more likely to appear earlier upon measurement. The non-dominant side will often appear weaker, and it is possible that the detection of the pulse will occur later than on the dominant side. The blood pressure on the dominant side can therefore appear to be higher than on the non-dominant side, although in reality they may be the same. In general, it could be said that a person tends to assert themselves through the dominant side of the body and that the non-dominant side has a withdrawn quality. This may have something to say about the aspects of the self that an individual does or doesn't express. The right side of the brain is concerned with emotion and may be the reason why there would be a deficiency pattern on the left hand side of the body. (Cozolino, 2006). It is accepted that blood pressure can vary between arms due to normal structural variations, but practice shows that the difference can be affected by the therapeutic intervention and the converse is true of the left handed, i.e. they tend to have a dominant left side.

Pathophysiological causes of right/left pulse differences:

- Arterial atheroma or aneurysm of the ascending aorto, supravascular aortic stenosis, subclavical steal syndrome, aortic arch syndrome (Llewelyn et al., 2006)

Temperature

There is a distinction between a physically abnormal body temperature and the abnormal experience of hot or cold. It is normal for the individual to be tolerant to a wide range of environmental temperature fluctuations and a dislike or aversion to hot and/or cold is often significant and indicative of imbalance.

Normal range: 36.6–37.2 C (98–99 F); fluctuates between individuals and there is also a diurnal variation within the individual, peaking in the evening and falling to a low in the early hours of the morning.

Oral: 36.8 C
Axilla: 36.4 C
Rectum: 37.3 C

Fever

Oral > 37.5 C; Rectal > 37.7 C

- Pathogenic invasion
- Hormone excess/deficiency

- Immunological reactions
- Inability to lose heat
- Malignancy
- Drug treatments

Hypothermia

< 35 C

- Lowered vital resistance (age, depletion)
- Hormone imbalance (e.g. myxoedema, pituitary)
- Drugs—recreational and treatment

A significant reduction in body temperature may indicate a pathological endocrine problem, e.g. hypothyroidism, however a small or moderate reduction may indicate a functional deficiency in the endocrine system. The main determinate of temperature is the metabolic rate and this is mainly determined by thyroxine. In a situation where there are significant depletion factors, the body may respond by endeavouring to conserve resources by lowering thyroid function and hence the metabolic rate. This would be in addition to other reductions in endocrine activity, e.g. adrenal cortical function and sympathetic autonomic activity.

Constitutional causes of sensorial experience of temperature

Cold

In the presence of a normal body temperature, cold may be experienced as peripheral cold with a normal feeling of body temperature or be experienced as a deep seated internal cold, which has a characteristic penetrating sensation to the core, 'I cannot get warm'. The significance is different, internal cold is the more serious expression of endocrine or energy depletion rather than an issue of blood circulation. Peripheral cold is related to the movement of blood and energy in relationship to the circulatory dynamics.

- Lowered vital resistance or reserve causing deficient energy and circulation—general or to a particular organ system, e.g. with general energy depletion, feeling of cold in the abdomen
- Stress—inhibition of the sympathetic nervous system
- Peripheral vasoconstriction causes cold hands, feet and head
- The patient may suffer from 'chilliphobia', i.e. an aversion to cold
- The patient may suffer from heat and cold in different modalities e.g. a cold exterior may lead to internal accumulation of heat
- Cold is often associated with, or leads to, hypofunction of an organ system

Cold externally is a manifestation of a withdrawal or negative response and is signified by cold symptoms and expression, e.g. cold hands and feet, pallor of the skin and the face in particular, a shrivelled expression. External cold signs and symptoms may signify internal heat patterns as cold and heat are interlinked and the colder the external expression, the hotter the internal dynamic may become. Complex interactions often exist, for example, someone with eczema, which is characterised by a hot internal reaction becoming externalised, may well have a constrictive nervous system pattern. A constrictive pattern creates a deficiency and hence cold reaction. An individual with heat in the blood may, therefore, feel hot and have hot hands but suffer from cold feet, i.e. the more proximal cold constriction is counteracted by the blood heat, but the distal cold constriction is not counteracted. Similarly, but for a different reason, menopausal women may be both hot and cold. The menopause often creates visceral constriction, which may manifest as hypertension, but at the same time there is a high level of heat, particularly during hot flushes. The constriction in the peripheral circulation actually prevents the diaphoresis of heat, creating a compressing action of the heat, which forces it upwards into the head and particularly the face, 'hectic cheeks' or 'mallor' flush. Although the woman feels intensely hot, symptomatically her skin may feel clammy, i.e. cold and damp not hot and dry, this is because of the action of the peripheral circulation.

Raynaud's disease is a vascular illness comprised of blood vessel spasm, particularly of the fingers and toes. It is a spinal reflex in response to changes in the ambient temperature and is not the same as the mechanisms that cause peripheral circulation. Primary Raynaud's is not related to underlying causes, but secondary Raynaud's is related to serious underlying inflammatory conditions, e.g. scleroderma, rheumatoid arthritis, lupus erythematosus. Symptoms can be mild or extremely painful and potentially serious.

Conflicting patterns of hot and cold are particularly apparent and important in the elderly. Endocrine depletion can cause both cold and hot reactions and the two may be closely linked. It is quite usual for an elderly person to be intolerant to both environmental heat and cold in an extreme way. This can be critical in the choice of herbal treatment as it is tempting to include the use of hot stimulating herbs in a situation of cold deficiency. This strategy might work well in a young person with a basically vital constitution, but could create an extreme heat overreaction in an elderly individual to the point where it could be life threatening.

Heat

In the presence of a normal body temperature the individual may experience heat permanently or at particular times of day or may become responsive to external or internal heat sources, e.g. hot ambient temperature, exercise, eating hot food and drinking hot drinks.

- Heat is often generated through hormone or endocrine deficiency, e.g. sex hormones, pancreatic, adrenal. Symptoms may be hot flushes or flashes. Deficiency of heat may be apparent through a mallor flush.
- Heat is often associated with toxic accumulation or faulty metabolism, but in most cases is concerned with immunological dysfunction and the accumulation of immune complexes.
- Liver heat may also connect with suppressed emotion, e.g. anger, resentment
- Heat may be symptomatic of a low grade pathogenic infection insufficient to manifest as fever, e.g. sub-acute cystitis.

- Heat expressed through a particular organ system may be significant of constitutional heat, e.g. recurrent sore throats, tonsillitis, may be an expression of heat in the system generally and will often worsen when the individual is under stress and therefore deficient. Deficiency causes an internalisation of function.
- The expression of heat may change its portal of expression, e.g. the development of cystitis in a patient being treated for eczema. The cystitis may in fact be an older disharmony, which is re-engaged by the intervention, i.e. a pattern of resolution invoking the historical progress of the condition.

Respiration

The number of respirations per minute under normal circumstances—16–22. There is a wide range of normal variations. Should be observed when the patient is unaware, e.g. whilst taking the pulse.

Tachypnoea

- Exercise
- Emotion and anxiety
- Fever
- Metabolic acidosis
- Hysterical over breathing

Facial colour

Facial colour and tone are consequences of the movement of blood and energy and hence to autonomic balance and activation.

- Pallor generally indicates deficiency of the peripheral circulation and is often associated with a condition of internal congestion. Pallor is frequently accompanied by other signs of circulatory deficiency, e.g. dark rings around or under the eyes. Pallor may also be indicative of blood quality problems.
- A condition of 'bright' paleness is indicative of active vasoconstriction, which occurs in conditions such as shock.
- Facial flushing or 'hectic' cheeks are generally indicative of hormone deficiency heat reaction and this may originate from a number of endocrine deficiency conditions.
- Swelling around the eyes, often dark in colour, is significant to fluid congestion and is generally related to liver and kidney function usually combined with fatigue factors.

Tongue diagnosis

Tongue diagnosis is of little significance in Western medicine, apart from the recognition of certain specific conditions.

- Glossitis is a condition where the tongue has a smooth and usually red surface due to atrophy of the papillae. This is generally a consequence of nutritional deficiencies, such as iron, folic acid or B vitamins, affecting the rapid mitosis of the mucosal cells. It is diagnostic of B12 deficiency.
- Pallor of the tongue and bucosal membranes is regarded as significant of anaemia but is not a reliable diagnostic measure.
- Lingua nigra is where the tongue has a black colouration due to the accumulation of keratin and is regarded to be symptomless and of unknown cause.
- Leucoplakia is a white coloured thickening of the mucosa of the tongue or mouth or of other membranes (anal, vaginal), which may be premalignant.
- The geographical tongue where the tongue has a cracked or lined appearance. It is not usually regarded as having any significance but can be a sign of vitamin B deficiency.

From the Eastern viewpoint, tongue diagnosis is of great significance in order to:

- Discern the pattern of disharmony, i.e. the functional disturbance and the organs involved.
- The severity of the disharmony, whether it is worsening or improving and the progress of the illness.
- As a sensitive and reliable indicator of internal changes.
- Provides an insight into internal dynamics, which is difficult to obtain via other techniques. The tongue is directly associated with the internal organs, notably the digestive tract and correspondingly shows changes to the associated tissues and circulation.

Important distinctions

- Chinese medical terminology is different to that of Western medicine and involves functional activity and movement in the concept of the organ systems. For example, the spleen in Chinese medicine refers to the organs of digestion, the process of digestion, the metabolism and transformation of food and relates to the fundamental state of energy.
- Qi refers to the energetic status, harmony or potential of the body or organ, yang to the active energy or function and yin to the state of the tissue integrity and nourishment.
- Tongue diagnosis must be considered in relation to the other signs and symptoms.
- Traditional Chinese patterns include pathologies that are extreme and refer to serious pathogenic infection, acute emergency or severe deficiency and are seldom seen in the practice of complementary practice in the West.
- Tongue diagnosis enables the practitioner to make a distinction between how the patient is and how he feels, i.e. it is an important indicator of tissue state.

Tongue examination

- Examine in good light, preferably natural light.
- Ask the patient to extend their tongue as far as possible but without strain as this can change the shape and colour of the tongue.

- The patient should not extend their tongue for more than 15–20 seconds, otherwise the colour may be affected. Repetitive extensions are permissible.
- The colour of the tongue may be affected by recently consumed food and drink or by medicines.

Characteristics of the tongue

Spirit or vitality

The colour and aspect of the tongue should be vibrant and vital in good health. It is significant to the prognosis of the condition, particularly the root.

Colour of the body

The colour of the body of the tongue is that which is underneath the coating, which may be a different colour and obscure the base. The normal colour is pale red. Colour is determined by the blood perfusion or quantitative flow of blood through the organ as a consequence of the circulatory dynamics and the balance of the ANS or is a reflection of the qualitative condition of the blood. Deficiency of blood results in paleness, which in Chinese medicine is a cold condition. Redness denotes a hot condition and may result from heat in the circulation or from lack of moisture to modify the red colour of the tongue. The base colour, therefore, shows hot and cold influences and is very indicative of the underlying circulatory, ANS and energy balances of the internal organs.

The tongue body may have raised papillae (points or spots); these are usually red but may be pale red, white or purple, and vary in size in different conditions. In general, papillae indicate heat, and their distribution on the tongue may be relevant to the organ systems affected. They may be the result of constitutional imbalance, e.g. deep anxiety or emotion or faulty food metabolism or as a consequence of exterior factors, such as the invasion of pathogens. Heat in different areas are referred to as particular organ systems in Chinese medicine, but care should be taken that these organs are not understandable as the same anatomical organs identified in the West. Heat in the anterior of the tongue, referred to as rising liver fire in Chinese medicine, often does have a clinical significance with inflammatory conditions associated with the throat, upper respiratory system or upper digestive system.

Shape

The normal tongue shape is neither too thin nor too swollen, is supple and without cracking. The consistency of the tongue is determined by the blood and moisture content. A thin tongue would therefore be considered too lacking in blood or moisture, as found in certain hormone deficiency states, and a swollen tongue would indicate a state of stagnation or congestion of the fluids (dampness) as found, for example, in sympathetic nerve deficiency. A swollen tongue may show crenulations where it presses against the teeth. Swelling in different areas of the tongue may suggest congestion in different organ systems.

Cracking in the tongue may be of different types and generally suggests heat, deficiency of moisture and restriction in circulation.

Coating

The tongue has a deep red, beefy colour, which is modified to its normal vital pink colour by a normal thin, white coating. The colour of the coating reflects hot or cold influences in the system; white coatings are significant of cold and yellow coatings are significant of heat. The thickness of the coating represents the extent of pathogenic factors. The coating is directly related to the mucous membranes of the upper digestive tract in particular and demonstrate the degree of mucous congestion present. In Chinese medicine the distribution of the coating signifies the organ systems involved, e.g. the more towards the root the coating is, the lower in the digestive tract the disharmony. There are conditions where the coating lifts from the base of the tongue to show shiny, red areas. This may indicate an underlying change in the trophic condition of the tongue membrane as a result of heat, hormone deficiency or nutritional deficiency.

Moisture

The normal tongue should be slightly moist, neither too dry nor too wet. Dryness may be a function of excess heat and when pronounced will lead to cracking of the tongue. Excess moisture may result from a general overactivity of the digestive process and be related to excess enzymatic secretion, including saliva.

Cracking

- Geographical tongue is an inherited and normal pattern of irregular cracking.
- Ice floe cracking: related to the impoverishment of moisture and trophic state of the tissues of the tongue consequent upon age-related depletion.
- Hormone deficiency cracking: a red, dry and cracked tongue caused by heat from hormone deficiency.
- A central crack or fissure: in physiological terms relates to energy depletion becoming significant at the tissue and organ level, i.e. a significant deterioration of foundational energy, but also relates to a poor sense of psychological foundation and sense of self.
- Cracking to the tip often relates to long standing emotional conflict, the emotional heart.

Case histories with analysis and interpretation

Case history: acne

This lady, aged 29, has acne to her cheeks and chin. The problem is continual but worsens when she is pre-menstrual. She has some hair growth on her chin and she has been investigated for polycystic ovarian syndrome (PCOS). Her energy is low, particularly in the mornings. She describes her mood as generally low and she describes herself as a worrier. She is hot at night. She has a headache once a week, particularly behind her right eye and she has migraines three or four times per year. Her menstrual cycle is three to three half weeks and she has significant pre-menstrual tension.

Clinical signs:
Blood pressure: 104/70. Pulse: 78.
Pulse pressure: 34. CVI: 13,572.
Tongue: red and swollen, yellow phlegm coating.

This lady is well presented, of normal weight, sociable and articulate. She lives with her partner. She is a fine artist. The historical, personal, and emotional circumstances of the patient were not disclosed or requested but her current life circumstances, in terms of her relationship with her partner and home and work situation, were described as happy. However, the low mood and anxiety suggest that there is a history of disharmony, which persists despite her current good psycho-social interconnection. In many ways having a good psycho-social environment is very helpful to the treatment intervention, as there are fewer obstacles to progress.

The clinical signs show a relatively low pulse pressure, this would give her symptoms of deficiency or disconnection. It is not clear to what extent the deficiency is a pattern of withdrawal or the result of fatigue factors and may be a combination of both.

Treatment rationale

The treatment intervention is aimed at nourishing foundational energy, which in addition to providing her with vitality will promote psychological well-being and sense of empowerment, strength and capacity. The movement towards externalisation, connection and manifestation will be enhanced by the Rosmarinus. The endogenous heat is further resolved with the triad of herbs, Schizandra, Iris and Rosa, with additional hepatic support from Glycyrrhiza and Paeonia.

Herb	Physiological actions	Energetic actions
Centella asiatica	Adaptogen. CNS and ANS regulator. Anti-inflammatory. Anxiolytic and antidepressant. (Gohil et al. 2010)	
Smilax	Foundational tonic and adaptogenic. Anti-inflammatory.	Sense of authority and foundation.
Schizandra asiatica	Adjunct for tonics and adaptogens.	Regulation of fire.
Iris	Liver tonic and adaptogen.	Expression of creativity and inspiration.
Rosa	Liver heat.	Resolution of emotional tension.
Glycyrrhiza	Nourishing foundational tonic.	Nourishment of self.
Paeonia	Liver restorative and clearance of heat.	Tranquillity. The inner 'beauty'.
Verbena	Nerve tonic and restorative.	Self-affirmation and strength.
Rosmarinus	ANS regulator.	Connection and manifestation of self.

Two weeks:
Blood pressure: 104/66.
Pulse 72.
Pulse pressure: 38.
Tongue: no phlegm coating, tongue is pale.

Improved energy, some improvement in the skin. Menstrual cycle four weeks. The patient wished for a more rapid improvement in her condition and so additional depurative herbs were added to the formula.

Arctium lappa seed	Bitter and resolvent for heat.
Plantago lanceolata	Demulcent. Depurative.

Six weeks:
Blood pressure: 100/58.
Pulse: 70.

Pulse pressure: 42.
Tongue: pink rather than red.

No headaches. Skin significantly improved.

Ten weeks:
Blood pressure: 104/62.
Pulse: 70.
Pulse pressure: 42.

The patient was happy with the outcomes, her skin was clear and she felt better energetically and with better mood and emotions and so she ceased treatment. The heat syndrome, as judged by the small amount of heat in the tongue, was not fully resolved, but there may be re-engagement with an intervention at a later date.

Case history: rheumatoid arthritis

This 47-year-old woman presented with a number of significant health problems but notably rheumatoid arthritis occurring in her small joints, which she has suffered from for some six years. She had a hysterectomy, two years previously, for heavy menstrual bleeding due to endometriosis. However, she continues to have a difficult hormone cycle, with fluid retention, significant mood disturbance and breast tenderness at the time when she would have been menstruating. She has a lymphangioma/pseudocyst in her abdomen which is thought to be congenital, but, is not currently causing any problems.

She has significant fatigue, especially in the winter. She suffers from the cold, which she feels invades her core, she has cold peripheral circulation and significant night sweats. She has chronic low grade sinus congestion and a history of sore throats.

Prescribed medications:
Methotrexate. Amitriptyline. Folic acid.
Supplements: Evening primrose oil. Vitamin C.

Clinical signs:
Blood pressure: 120/80.
Pulse: 94.
Pulse pressure: 40.
CVI: 18,800.
Tongue: widespread, deep cracking, pale centre with heat to the tip and edges.

This lady is fashionably dressed, well-groomed and of normal weight. She is communicative, articulate and sociable. She is married to her second husband and has one son. She has had a history of turbulent relationships and family problems, although she is now in a steady and harmonious relationship. A very significant event in her timeline was the death of her sister from cancer. She had a very close relationship with her sister and she was particularly distraught that her sister's children were left without their mother.

This lady feels 'fragile', fragmented and extremely depleted. The aims of the intervention are to nourish a stronger foundation and improve her immune system and the associated heat and inflammation. The process of authentication, nourishment and healing will enable her to come to terms with her deep emotional wounds.

Herb	Dosage	Actions
Achillea millefolium	15.00	Circulatory facilitator and regulator for the circulation.
Astragalus membraneous	15.00	Foundational tonic and immunological facilitator and regulator.
Centella asiatica	15.00	CNS and ANS balancer and regulator. Anti-inflammatory.
Smilax ornata	20.00	Foundational tonic. Anabolic agent. Anti-inflammatory and alterative.
Schizandra chinensis	10.00	Adjunct for tonic actions. Regulation of the 'fire' principle.
Guaiacum officinale	15.00	Dispersive alterative and anti-inflammatory.
Articum lappa seed	15.00	Intense dispersing alterative.
Plantago lanceolata	15.00	Soothing, demulcent, tissue healing.
Rosa damacena	10.00	Resolution of liver heat. Transformative agent for emotional tension.
Vitex agnus castus	15.00	Pituitary hormone regulator.
Anemone pulsatilla	10.00	Hormone regulator. Facilitator for psycho-social boundaries.
	155.00	

Four weeks:
Blood pressure: 110/72.
Pulse: 88.
Pulse pressure: 38.
Tongue: reduced heat, pinker in the centre.

Little hormonal disturbance with slight breast pain for two days only. General improvement in energy and well-being and increased feeling of appreciation of life.

Twelve months:
Blood pressure: 102/64.
Pulse: 86.
Pulse pressure: 38.
CVI: 14,276.

No inflammation. General improvement in energy and well-being and has now sufficient energy to carry out exercise. Blood tests show slightly low neutrophil count, ESR is within normal levels. Has been slowly reducing methotrexate medication.

Case history: chronic sinus congestion

This 36-year-old mother of two complains a of chronic sinus condition which gives her considerable pain. She has a history of recurrent tonsillitis and sore throats since childhood and the sinus condition has been present since the age of 11. She has tried dietary manipulation, including dairy free, to no avail. Anti-histamines do not affect it.

She feels generally fatigued and lethargic. She is hot during the day and night but has cold feet. Her systems are normal. The patient is sociable, articulate and confident. She says that she is sensitive, inclined to feel tense, but not anxious. She reports that her life generally is relatively unproblematic.

Clinical signs:
Blood pressure: 120/84.
Pulse: 84.
Pulse pressure: 36.
CVI: 17,136.

Analysis and interpretation:
This lady has an autonomic dysregulation, which stems from her childhood. The pulse pressure is low, demonstrating a significant deficiency state but her CVI is relatively high due to a high pulse rate, which is probably compensating for the low pulse pressure. As a consequence, her blood perfusion is poor, which is shown in the pale tongue base. There is no history of anaemia, as demonstrated by blood tests, which supports the diagnosis of a quantitative blood deficiency. This is a cold pattern, although the endogenous heat shown in the anterior of the tongue, renders her sensorial experience as one of heat. She is hot in the day and especially at night but has cold feet. The reason for this is that the heat pattern overcomes the cold deficiency pattern, but not for the feet which are at the distal end of the circulation. The diastolic blood pressure is somewhat elevated and suggests a pattern of smooth muscle constraint, which for someone of her age, would normally be reflective a level of psychogenic tension. This is typical to someone of a sensitive nature, the tendency to be aroused and overwhelmed by sensorial information, emotionality and stimulation. The combination of sympathetic deficiency and smooth muscle restriction leads to excess visceral activation and consequently hyperaemia, congestion and mucous secretion of the membranes. The phlegm and membrane congestion are the main cause of the sinus problem. A phlegm coating is visible on the tongue and is reflective of the mucus problem extending throughout the mucous membranes, including the digestive tract, although it is only symptomatically present in the sinuses.

Herb	Dosage	Actions
Centella asiatica	15.00	CNS and ANS balance and regulation.
Smilax ornata	20.00	Foundational and anabolic tonic.
Schizandra chinensis	10.00	Tonic adjunct and heat circulation.

(Continued)

Herb	Dosage	Actions
Hydrastis canadensis	15.00	Membrane tissue astringent and restorative. Alterative for liver heat.
Althaea Officinalis herba	30.00	Soothing membrane demulcent and restorative. Aids the resolution of heat reassuring.
Rosa damacena	10.00	Soothing and reassuring for liver heat and emotionality connected to heat.
Hyssopus officinalis	15.00	Autonomic and nervine regulator.
Stachys betonica	20.00	Autonomic and cerebral circulatory regulator.
Rosmarinus officinalis	15.00	Authentication and manifestation of self.
Dosage: 5 ml bid aq ac.	150.00	

Case history: hypertension

This lady, aged 48, presents with free floating anxiety and a long history of hypertension. She describes herself as hypervigilant, 'head orientated' and with a driven personality. She describes her energy as poor unless she is actively engaged in a work pursuit. She reacts to red wine and chocolate with a heat reaction and palpitations. She also suffers from attacks of palpitations at other times. Headaches are rare but she does have significant neck and shoulder tension. Her head is clear and she would describe herself as 'present'. Her core is hot and she has significantly cold extremities, especially her feet. She has IBS, notably an inclination to loose stools, wind and turbulence.

She has had amenorrhoea for four years and considers herself as now through the menopause. She started a low dose HRT two years ago, which she thought helped, but she is keen to stop this. She has a distaste for orthodox medication.

Context:
This lady is clearly intelligent, self-aware and insightful. She is conventionally and smartly dressed and well-groomed. She is sociable and articulate. She seems agitated and sensitive. She is married and has no children.

Supplements: Vitamin D3 4000 i.u., vitamin B complex, fish oil.

Clinical signs:
Blood pressure: 164/100.
Pulse: 82.
Pulse pressure: 64.
CVI: 21,648.
Tongue: swollen, generalised heat.

Key therapeutic actions:
Embodiment. Sense of self. Control.

Therapeutic analysis:
This lady has a significant sympathetic excess pattern as indicated by her relatively high systolic blood pressure, raised pulse pressure and relatively fast pulse rate together with her feeling of being vigilant. The excess pattern is partly understandable by the pattern of constraint shown by her high diastolic blood pressure as this would need a significant compensatory rise in cardiac output. Other considerations are the consequences of hormone deficiency following the menopause and also depletion factors. It is significant that her energy profile is poor when she is not sympathetically activated, i.e. not at work. Adrenal fatigue would contribute to an early menopause. It would appear that she is operating via an adrenally activated system rather than a serotonergic. This could be a consequence of a number of factors, i.e. poor energy foundation, low sense of self and self-esteem and vigilance from the need to control her boundaries.

Pathophysiological considerations:
There is a possibility of cardiovascular disease with an increased cardiovascular output to compensate for a compromised tissue state.
    Anaemia. Increased cardiovascular output could be compensatory for poor blood quality.
    Hypertension may be a cause or consequence of liver or kidney disease.
    Metabolic syndrome.

Herbal intervention

Herb	Dosage	Physiological actions	Energetic actions
Angelica archangelica spagyric	10.00	Spasmolytic.	Protective. Sense of calm and safety.
Centela asiatica	15.00	CNS. ANS regulator. Tonic. Adaptogen.	The great organiser.
Codonopsis pilosa	20.00	Foundation tonic. Adaptogen.	Sense of authority and control. Foundation.
Lycium	10.00	Tonic for the liver, pancreas and adrenals.	Sweet and nourishing.
Agrimonia eupatoria	10.00	Astringent. Bitter. Liver and digestive tonic.	Resolvent. Facilitates the process of acceptance.
Taraxacum off. radix	20.00	Foundational tonic. Liver restorative. Hepatic.	Grounding. Establishment of sense of self.
Polygonum multif	20.00	Tonic. Adaptogen.	Nourishes foundational energy.
Stachys betonica	20.00	Cerebral and nervine tonic.	Autonomic regulation and interconnection.

(Continued)

Herbal intervention (Continued)

Herb	Dosage	Physiological actions	Energetic actions
Rosamarinus off.	10.00	ANS balancer. Restorative. Aromatic.	Being manifest.
Viola odourata	15.00	Lymphatic and depurative.	Promotes presentation of self and self-worth.
	150.00		

Rationale:
This patient is functioning very effectively in her psycho-social environment and has developed refined qualities to enable working at a high level of communication and conceptual understanding. She is also clearly 'sensitive' in her appreciation, recognising the beauty and intrinsic value of things. She does not, however, feel safe and feels the need to police her boundaries continuously. The medicine is designed to embody her by bringing her into a closer relationship with herself and to improve her sense of integration. The patient also needs significant physiological nourishment and support.

Prognosis:
It is anticipated that the patient will make a slow transformation from being 'head orientated' to being 'core orientated'. This process will be accompanied by a growing sense of self and self-esteem. The need for vigilance and guarding will diminish and hence the systolic and diastolic blood pressures will decrease. The process needs to be slow and steady.

Two weeks:
Blood pressure: 156/100.
Pulse: 80.

Experienced an acute viral infection

Seven weeks:
Blood pressure: 152/98.
Pulse: 76.

Eleven weeks:
Blood pressure: 150/98.
Pulse: 80.

The patient is no longer feeling vigilant but feels empty and vacuous with a sense of disorientation and lack of control. She has experienced disturbed sleep with bizarre dreams.

Six months:
Blood pressure: 140/90.
Pulse: 70.
Pulse pressure: 50.
CVI: 16,100.

The patient is showing a very significant improvement in cardiovascular function, the pulse pressure and pulse are normal, however, there is still some elevation of the diastolic blood pressure. The patient is well but wishes to continue to improve her diastolic blood pressure and ideally achieving a target of a diastolic pressure of 80. The tongue shows some generalised heat with more pronounced heat in the tip. The tongue is swollen with significant scalloping.

Case history: enlarged right ventricle

This lady, aged 70, was diagnosed with an enlarged right ventricle eight years ago and wishes to seek treatment to improve her cardiovascular health. She has some shortness of breath but otherwise is symptom free. She describes her energy as poor, especially in the late afternoon. Her head is clear but she has some problems with her memory. She has cold peripheral circulation.

Clinical signs:
Blood pressure: 120/80.
Pulse: 74. Pulse pressure: 40.
CVI: 14,560.
Pulse character: deep, strong, fluctuating.

Context:
The patient describes herself as a determined, self-motivated and independent woman, however, she has had a number of close relationships with domineering men which have left her feeling emotionally compromised, particularly a relationship that ended some eight years ago. She has trained as a Steiner teacher. She is clearly insightful, emotionally intelligent and highly articulate.

Analysis:
The clinical signs show a degree of deficiency with a pulse that is compensatory, giving a slightly high CVI. There is some degree of constraint in the circulation.

Herb	Dosage	Actions
Angelica archangelica radix	10.00	Aromatic circulatory stimulant and relaxant. Female tonic.
Centella asiatica	15.00	ANS and CNS regulator. Tonic restorative. Anti-inflammatory.
Eleutherococcus sentinosus	20.00	Foundational tonic and adaptogen.

(Continued)

Herb	Dosage	Actions
Schizandra chinensis	10.00	Adjunct for tonics and adaptogens. The movement of 'fire'.
Iris versicolor	15.00	Liver tonic and adaptogen. Promotion of female creativity and inspiration.
Rosa damacena	10.00	Liver heat. Resolution of emotional anger and frustration.
Glycyrrhiza glabra	15.00	Nourishing foundational tonic.
Stachys betonica	20.00	Autonomic.
Verbena officinalis	10.00	Nerve tonic and restorative. Self-affirmation and belief.
Salvia triloba	10.00	Autonomic and hormone regulator.
Crataegus fructus	15.00	Heart regulator. Cardiovascular tissue restorative.
Dosage: 5 ml bid.	150.00	

Week	Blood pressure	Pulse	Pulse pressure	CVI	
0	120/80	74	40	14,560	
2	110/76	80	34	14,880	Feeling stronger.
6	112/66	70	42	12,460	Four weeks of viral type infection with copious phlegm.
10	118/68	72	46	13,392	Autonomic balance improved and so the emphasis was placed on energy foundation. Borago and Polygonum replaced Stachys and Glycyrrhiza.
15	124/68	64	56	12,288	

The patient disclosed that she felt more manifest, more 'herself', speaking her mind. Stronger and more energetic. The patient recognised that the 'viral' infection she acquired after the first few weeks was a process of physiological and psychological catharsis and when this had cleared she made significant progress. Her consultant is of the opinion that her heart condition is stable and no further treatment is required.

Case history: disconnection

The patient presented with a feeling of disconnection. She said that she felt like a bird being kept in a cage and she wanted to be free to spread her wings and fly. She feels 'full of crap', doubtful about her life choices, apart from motherhood, which she regards as her saviour.

The patient feels 'scatty' in her head, muzzy-headed and disconnected. She has tight shoulders and burning in her spine. She describes her energy as poor and herself as physically and emotionally drained and unsupported. Her digestion is turbulent and inclined to wind and bloating. She has occasional acid indigestion. She tends to have hypoglycaemia and feels that she really needs to eat but doesn't feel like eating or know what to eat. She has cold peripheral circulation. Her menstrual cycle was previously very heavy but it is much improved since the Mirena coil was fitted.

Context:
The patient is the mother of two children, 7 and 10, who is separated from her partner and father of the children. She has an acrimonious relationship with the father who she claims uses the children as a means of aggression against her. She is legally obliged to permit him to share access but is of the opinion that he bullies them. She has no support.

Clinical signs:
Blood pressure: 123/59.
Pulse: 62.
Pulse pressure: 64.
Tongue: pale and swollen with superficial heat.

Analysis:
The clinical signs show a normal diastolic blood pressure and a slightly elevated systolic giving a pulse pressure of 62. This may be compensatory for a slightly low pulse. The low pulse might reflect a slow metabolism and the possibility of subclinical hypothyroidism, perhaps secondary to endocrine depletion.

The patient would appear to be in a classic entanglement. A key factor in her situation may be an impairment in her capacity to implement effective decision-making. This is often the consequence of being raised in an environment of compliance with adult authority and may lead to entering controlling relationships. She is unable to manifest the important requirements in her life, and is therefore dependent upon others, and as a consequence is resentful and angry. She is unable to find suitable employment, her benefits provide little money, she is in considerable debt and unable to pay her rent and has few supporters.

The herbal intervention is designed for physiological nourishment and to provide the strength to deal with her circumstances. Although she is intelligent and well educated with good interpersonal skills she would appear to lack the core personal facilities of strong self-belief, personal esteem and the capacity for good decision making.

Herb	*Physiological actions*	*Energetic actions*
Anemone pulsatilla	Spasmolytic. Nervine.	Protection and openness.
Centella asiatica	ANS and CNS regulation.	Control and regulation.
Panax quinqufolium	Tonic. Adaptogen.	Regulation. Synthesis of the male and female.
Lycium	Adjunct for tonification.	Regulation of 'fire'.
Iris versicolor	Hepatic. Bitter.	Promotion of feminine creativity and insight.
Paeonia laterifolium	Liver restorative.	Sense of beauty.

(*Continued*)

Herb	Physiological actions	Energetic actions
Glycyrrhiza glabra	Demulcent. Foundational tonic. Depurative.	
Taraxacum officinale radix	Liver restorative and tonic.	Sense of self.
Arctium lappa radix	Liver restorative and tonic.	Sense of self.
Verbena officinale	Nervine tonic and restorative.	Self-belief and affirmation.
Rosa damacena	Nerve tonic. Heat.	Emotional resolution.
Salvia triloba	ANS regulator.	Sense of individuation and self-regulation.

Three months:
Blood pressure: 130/80.
Pulse: 88.

The patient has a notable increase in diastolic blood pressure and the patient commented that she had started to feel emotionally uncomfortable and tense, which she ascribed to becoming more connected to her emotions as opposed to feeling dissociated.

Six months:
Blood pressure: 112/70.
Pulse: 70.
Pulse pressure: 42.

The patient described herself as more self-contained, independent and assured. She has good legal support, the support of a social work agency with a dedicated co-worker and she has now entered employment. She no longer required herbal treatment.

Case history: stress

This man, aged 40, is a company director of a family firm. He presented with a post-traumatic stress condition following an episode of acute stress and a stay in a residential crisis centre. He feels anxious and disorientated. His energy levels are described as low but says that he is driven in his work and life style. He has a long history of using alcohol as self-medication. He wishes to seek a different 'mindset', a more Zen in approach, and to develop a stronger sense of self. He has started studying and exploring self-development practices. He has a cold periphery and nocturnal heat. His head feels cloudy. He feels disconnected.

Clinical signs:
Blood pressure: 112/76.
Pulse: 86.

Pulse pressure: 36.
Tongue: swollen, heat in the tip, phlegm coating to the rear.

Analysis:
The clinical signs show a deficiency pattern, with a low systolic output, low pulse pressure and some diastolic tension with a compensatory increased pulse rate. The pattern is reflected in the tongue with a pale, swollen base, heat in the tip and phlegm congestion to the rear. The patient is at a critical time in his life when he needs to develop his sense of personal autonomy and strength in order to break free of his constraints and undergo life changing decisions.

Herb	Dosage	Physiological actions	Energetic actions
Angelica archangelica radix	15.00	Circulatory regulator.	Facilitation of good boundaries.
Panax ginseng	15.00	Core foundational tonic.	Core strength and integrity.
Astragalus membraneous	15.00	Foundational and immuno-regulatory tonic.	Builds the capacity to assert and police one's self.
Schizandra chinensis	10.00	Adjunct for tonics.	Circulates the 'fire' principle.
Agrimonia eupatorium	15.00	Liver tonic and astringent.	Resolution of liver heat.
Taraxacum officinalis radix	20.00	Foundational tonic.	Fosters 'sense of self'.
Borago officinalis	20.00	Adrenal tonic.	
Stachys betonica	30.00	Autonomic regulator. Cerebral-spinal restorative.	
Rosmarinus	15.00	Autonomic regulator.	Manifestation of self.
Flower essences: Agrimony. Cherry Plum. Walnut		Facilitators for change: Acceptance. Trust. Freedom.	
	155.00		

Four weeks:
Blood pressure: 120/70.
Pulse: 86. Pulse pressure: 50.
Tongue: slight heat in the tip.

Energy is reported as improved. Sleep improved. Less revved. Less hot.

Herbs for integration and harmony

Rosacea (Rose family)

Roses represent femininity, grace, beauty, love and affection, free spirit, clarity. Most of the members of the Rose family share the capacity to bring these qualities forward and to resolve and heal emotional trauma, turmoil and tensions. The colour rose in esoteric terms represents the ray of love and devotion and brings this psycho-spiritual force into manifestation. Rose may be included in formulations in its manifestation in the different species which have a particular resonance to an organ system.

- Crataeus—heart
- Rubus—uterus
- Potentilla—digestion
- Agrimonia—liver
- Prunus—lungs
- Rosa—nervous system
- Alchemilla arvensis—urinary tract
- Alchemilla vulgaris—uterus
- Filipendula—upper digestive tract

Lamiaceae (Labiatae)

A family with many medicinal plants some of which have very distinctive features. Some have a representation to assist with the expression of self. Physiologically this is a combination of stimulation, relaxation and toning creating a balance of the autonomic nervous system and optimal well-being and balance. Salvia, Rosmarinus and Hyssopus are particularly relevant to the manifestation of self, i.e. being fully present in the world and having a sense of being connected.

Boraginaceae

The Borage family contain a number of important herbs, which are active in promoting tissue healing and cellular replication. Esoterically the healing actions are said to apply also to the fragmentation of energy vibration that underlies tissue damage, e.g. shock.
Different species relate to particular organ systems.

- Borago—adrenal restoration
- Symphytum—connective tissues
- Pulmonaria—lungs

Herb	Therapeutic movement and actions	Conditions applicable and combinations	Energetic actions and notes
Aletris farionosa	Bitter. Stimulating and relaxing. Tonic. Endocrine agent.	Female tonic. Dysmenorrhoea. Uterine prolapse.	Opens and aligns sexuality but in the Goddess sense. Sensuality and sexuality integrated with femininity and love. The self-actualised woman in the corporeal self.
Arctium lappa root and seed	Depurative. Restorative. Harmonising. Soothing. Seed is a bitter and penetrating alterative.	Wide acting depurative. Trophorestorative for the liver and kidneys. Seed is specific for rising endogenous heat reactions especially affecting the head-acne, eczema, furunculosis.	Integrative and restorative.
Citrus aurantium flores	Warm. Moist. Sweet. Bitter. Antidepressant. Sedative. Antispasmodic. Carminative. Astringent. Bitter and cholagogue. Antiseptic.	Mood elevator. Insomnia. Sedative and spasmolytic for anxiety, tension and associated symptoms, e.g. nervous headache, dyspepsia.	Helps ease emotional tension. A good facilitator.

(*Continued*)

Herb	Therapeutic movement and actions	Conditions applicable and combinations	Energetic actions and notes
		Hypertension and palpitations. Clears heat from the liver and associated organs. **Special features: a strong and uplifting tranquilliser**.	
Hypericum perforatum	Cool. Dry. Bitter. Astringent. Relaxing, restorative. Nerve tonic. Antidepressant. Antibacterial. Antiviral. Anti-inflammatory. Vulnerary. Antihaemorrhagic. Liver restorative.	Relaxing and tonic for anxiety, restlessness, depression, insomnia. Shock. Nerve injuries. Antispasmodic for GIT and genitourinary tract. Antiviral action against: Herpes 1 and 2, zoster. Epstein Barr etc. Reduces prolactin production. Topical—burns, blisters, wounds, tumours, herpes.	Esoterically associated with protection during spiritual transition and a harbinger of spiritual change.
Hyssopus officinale	Stimulant. Relaxant. Sedative. Antiviral. Antispasmodic. Anti-inflammatory. Diaphoretic. Expectorant. Antitussive. Affinity for the throat and lungs.	Specifically 'nervine', stimulating and relaxing for ANS balancing. Purification. The transformation of negative energy patterns. Protection. Affirming for self.	Releases deep seated tension and disharmony.
Iris versicolor	Cool. Dry. Bitter. Astringent Sweet. Anti-inflammatory.	Physiologically a discharging liver herb for liver heat: eczema, psoriasis, acne.	In Greek mythology Iris is the personification of the rainbow. As the sun links heaven and earth, Iris links the gods to humanity.

(Continued)

Herb	Therapeutic movement and actions	Conditions applicable and combinations	Energetic actions and notes
	Lymphatic, hepatic depurative. Tissue astringent and purifier.	Migraine and headache of liver origin. Endogenous heat invading the throat, i.e. chronic sore throats, thyroiditis.	She is the personification of the female creative inspiration and inherent beauty. Energetically releases creativity and openness by opening a portal to the ethereal self through the liver channel.
Lavendula angustifolia	Cool. Dry. Bitter. Pungent. Dispersing, stimulating restoring. Antidepressant. Relaxant. Sedative. Carminative. Stimulant. Cholagogue,. choleretic. Antirheumatic.	Anxiety, depression. nervous irritability, insomnia. Spasm congestion associated with the GIT—colic, bloating, IBS. Nausea and vomiting. Motion sickness. Cerebral insufficiency— headache, migraine, memory, vertigo. Antineoplastic. Topical—anti-inflammatory, insect bites, dermatological agent, rubefacient, vulnerary, burns, neuralgia, strains and bruises. **Special features: balancing to the ANS—stimulates, relaxes and calms.**	Works on the higher CNS centres. For disharmony from shock and other invasion. General facilitator.
Matricaria chamomilla/ Chamaemelum nobile	Cooling or warming. Calming. Bitter. Astringent.	Anxiety, restlessness, insomnia. Antispasmodic for the GIT, respiratory and genitourinary systems. Headaches and migraines.	

(Continued)

HERBS FOR INTEGRATION AND HARMONY

Herb	Therapeutic movement and actions	Conditions applicable and combinations	Energetic actions and notes
	Antispasmodic. Sedative. Anti-inflammatory. Antibacterial. Antifungal. Diaphorectic. Aromatic	Allergic reactions and membrane inflammation—respiratory, digestive, genital. Nausea and vomiting. Motion sickness. Amenorrhoea. Dysmenorrhoea. Eczema, dermatitis, impetigo, insect bites, burns, wounds. Teething pains, earache etc. in children. **Special features: antispasmodic and ani-inflammatory for all systems.** Children's complaints.	
Ocimum basiculum			
Pelargonium graveolens	Cool. Moist. Clears heat and inflammation. Antidepressant. Astringent. Anti-inflammatory. Haemostatic. Vulnerary. Aphrodisiac. Tonic.	Uplifting and relaxing for anxiety and depression, stress. Emotional tension associated with hormonal states—PMT, menopause. Aphrodisiac and adrenal tonic. Astringent for diarrhoea. Topical for sore throats as a gargle. Eczema. **Special features: uplifting relaxant that has a restorative and nourishing action.**	

(*Continued*)

Herb	Therapeutic movement and actions	Conditions applicable and combinations	Energetic actions and notes
Prunella vulgaris	Antioxidant. Wound healing. Antibacterial. Anti-tumour. Astringent. Hypotensive.	Wound healing. Haematuria. Hypertension.	In esoteric terms, connects the person to their deep, inherent capacity to self-heal.
Rosa spp. damascena	Cold. Dry. Clears heat. Restores and nourishes. Antidepressant. Sedative. Astringent. Anti-inflammatory. Hepatic, cholagogue. Anticholesterolaemic. Aphrodisiac. Antipyretic. Antiviral.	Relaxing and uplifting for anxiety and depression. Cleansing, tonic and restorative to the liver. Clears liver and blood heat—eczema, dermatitis. Menorrhagia, metrorrhagia, uterine fibroids. Hormonally associated emotional upset. Depression. Aphrodisiac. Fertility enhancer. Antiviral agent, HIV. Laxative especially for children. Astringent and anti-inflammatory for mouth ulcers, gingivitis, conjunctivitis. Topical—radiation burns, dermatitis.	A key regulator for the emotional heart.
Rosmarinus officinalis	Bitter. Pungent. Aromatic. Stimulating, relaxing, restorative, resolving. Relaxant. Metabolic stimulant. Diaphoretic. Affinity for the digestion.	Circulating and restorative for the peripheral and cerebral circulation. Digestive deficiency conditions. Headache from deficiency. Circulatory weakness. Adaptogenic.	Being manifest, 'presence' and the expression of one's self. Specific for regulation of the digestive function. Connection with life—becoming manifest. Protection.

(Continued)

Herb	Therapeutic movement and actions	Conditions applicable and combinations	Energetic actions and notes
		Adrenal tonic. Antiseptic and immune enhancing.	
Salvia off. See also: Salvia trilobal, Salvia sclarea, Salvia miltiorrhiza (Dan Shen).	Tonic. Nervine restorative. Adrenal trophorestorative. Astringent. Aromatic. Stimulant. Relaxant. Antispasmodic. ANS balancer. Antibioltic. Antifungal. Antiviral. Antiseptic. Anti-inflammatory. Hormone balancer. Affinity for the head.	Endocrine stimulant and restorative. Anxiety, depression. Debility and weakness. Bacterial, viral, fungal infection. Immunostimulating. Tonsillitis, laryngitis, pharyngitis, gingivitis. Hormone imbalance. Infertility. Improves cerebral circulation. Hyperhydrosis. Sexual dysfunction—hyper or hypo. Suppresses prolactin release. Hot flushes and menopausal sweats and hormonal disturbances at menopause.	Endocrine agent. CNS and ANS balancer. Sympathetic restorative. Conditions of congestion, infection and inflammation associated with the head and upper digestive tract. Psycho-spiritual regulation and control.
Scutellaria laterifolia	Cold. Dry. Bitter. Astringent. Antispasmodic. Sedative. Nerve. Tonic. Anti-inflammatory. Anodyne. Anticonvulsant.	Nervous restlessness, excitability, panic, anxiety, insomnia, obsession. Nerve restorative for weak, debilitated, sensitive systems. Deliriuim tremens. Hysteria. Epilepsy. Convulsions. Muscular spasms and tremors. Hypertension.	Particularly effective for working with anxiety associated with deep patterns of trauma.

(Continued)

Herb	Therapeutic movement and actions	Conditions applicable and combinations	Energetic actions and notes
		Clears heat and toxins from the liver and kidneys. **Special features: a relaxing and sedating herb with long term benefits of tonification and strengthening**.	
Stachys betonica	Cold. Dry. Bitter. Astringent. Scatters wind heat. Tonic. Antispasmodic. Cerebral stimulant. Alterative. Astringent. Hepatic.	Cerebral tonic and restorative—memory, concentration, headache, vertigo. Eye problems from deficiency—cataract, conjunctivitis, poor eye sight. Anxiety. Panic attacks. GIT relaxant and tonic. Cleansing action on the liver—rheumatism, sciatica. Astringent, healing action on mucous membranes. Diarrhoea. Haemostatic. Vulnerary. **Special features: a relaxing and stimulating herb that removes toxaemia and stasis from the viscera and encourages the upward and outward flow of blood and energy. Has long-term regenerative action.**	Enables a connection and expression to be made between emotional repressions and conscious experience.

(Continued)

Herb	Therapeutic movement and actions	Conditions applicable and combinations	Energetic actions and notes
Taraxacum officinale radix	Bitter liver tonic and restorative. Cholagogue. Diuretic. Detoxicant.	Liver disorders. Cholelithiasis but where obstructed. Pancreatic disorders. Anorexia and indigestion.	Foundational tonic for the establishment of the 'sense of self'. The father 'archetype'.
Verbena officinalis	Cool. Dry. Bitter. Astringent. Eliminative. Restorative. Diffusive. ANS Relaxant Tonic. Bitter. Cholagogue. Diaphoretic. Antidepressant. Emmenagogue. Galactagogue.	Spasmodic nervine and antidepressant for debilitated nervous conditions. Anxiety, insomnia, irritability. Stimulant and tonic to the liver, gall bladder and GIT, removing heat and toxicity. Antispasmodic for asthma, bronchitis, sinus problems. Amenorrhoea, dysmenorrhoea—tones and cleanses the uterus. Urinary tract spasm, dysuria, gravel. Aphrodisiac. **Special features: relaxing, cleansing, astringing tonic for the viscera—removing obstructions and facilitating a diffusive and externalising action**.	For the tension and scattered disharmony associated with over striving, anxiety and competitiveness. Facilitator for change. The pure resonance of purple, which is the perfect blend of red and blue, i.e. action and insight.
Viola spp.	Bitter. Cooling. Anti-inflammatory. Depurative. Hepatic. Lymphatic.		A particular representation or quality of Viola is to be undiscovered or overlooked, they are so easily passed by,

(Continued)

Herb	Therapeutic movement and actions	Conditions applicable and combinations	Energetic actions and notes
			but they also can be very present. When you see them emerge they are beautiful, alive and poignant. In this sense they have the capability of moving between overt and covert. They are therefore very helpful in developing a sophisticated relationship between the self and the world. Viola odourata could be seen as more suitable for harmonising the internal emotional dynamics, and Viola tricolour for harmonising the relationship of the internal emotional dynamic with the psycho-social environment.
Viscum album	Cold. Moist. Antispasmodic. Sedative. Tonic. Hypotensive. Haemostatic.	Relaxant for anxiety, tension, panic attacks. Antispasmodic for hypertension. Cardiac tonic. Immune stimulant. Uterine stimulant and antihemorrhagic (post-partum). **Special features: reduces excess parasympathetic nerve activity**. Antidepressant withdrawal.	For the release of emotional constraint.

Prescribing

> Thoughts give birth to a creative force that is neither elemental nor sidereal. Thoughts create a new heaven, a new firmament, a new source of energy, from which new arts flow. When a man undertakes to create something, he establishes a new heaven, as it were, and from it the work that he desires to create flows into him. For such is the immensity of man that he is greater than heaven and earth.
>
> (Paracelsus, in Ball, 2006)

Intention

The medicine only does what it is designed to do. The implication of this is that the designer needs to have a very clear and specific will for the intention behind the design of the medicine. This does not mean necessarily having an expectation of a specific outcome, it can be non-specific, e.g. to enhance the self-esteem of the patient. Here we mean will as thought and feeling. It is useful to consider the difference between personal or mind will and what has been called soul will. A prescription could be regarded as an act of creation and the creative act is in the formulation of the prescription, not in the dispensing. Although we think in a linear process of cause and effect, in reality the impact of the medicine is much more global and complex. The patient may have a condition that they regard as the priority for treatment but following a discussion regarding the more underlying aspects of the case it can be helpful to have a set of intentions for the outcome agreed between the patient and practitioner. Examples would be sense of freedom, embodiment, self-belief, vitality. These are more general outcomes that the patient can clearly understand and encompass.

Faith is that 'authority comes from certainty and certainty comes from self-belief', i.e. know what it is that you are endeavouring to do and believe and trust in it. Self-belief on the part of the practitioner is essential.

The science of prescribing

Prescribing can be deemed to be a scientific process comprised of the following elements.

The problem—the presenting complaint.

Gathering data on the complaint; the clinical signs and symptoms and the context gained from the case history.

Interpretation and analysis of the data to understand the process of the complaint.

A hypothesis to explain the situation.

A treatment plan: usually involving a herbal intervention.

The prognosis to indicate what would be expected in terms of changes in signs and symptoms and the patient's experience, which would need to be demonstrated in order to uphold the hypothesis.

Assessment of the outcome in terms of the signs and symptoms and the patient's experience. This would include effective decision-making and behaviour responses on behalf of the patient.

Active v passive engagement of the patient

Traditionally the patient has a passive engagement with medicines, i.e. the medicine has a direct physiological action with which the patient has little engagement with psychologically, although clearly the patient can modify the action and help or hinder its effects. This is primarily a quantitative intervention and so the physical attributes of the medicine and the dosage are relevant and important. Physiologically directed medicines tend to remain physiological. Conversely the patient could have an active engagement with medicines. This means that the medicine changes the way in which the patient themselves respond to a situation. This is a psycho-physiological action in which the patient is empowered and takes more responsibility. In this sense the attributes necessary in the medicine are whatever it takes to activate the patient's response and are likely to be variable and individually specific. The medicine is more likely to be qualitative and representational, as it is acting upon the affective and sensorial modalities of the patient.

Reassurance v self-actualisation

The patient may seek reassurance and be grateful to receive it, but this does not necessarily lead to an internal psycho-physiological change that enables the patient to become empowered and make good decisions in their best interests. Self-actualisation of the self might be a desirable outcome, but there must be congruence between the expectations of the patient and the practitioner. There can be a danger of the practitioner being focussed on their own outcomes, which they are acting out through the patient–practitioner interaction. The patient outcomes are more important than those of the practitioner and need to be determined. It is essential that an agreement is reached between the patient and the practitioner about the purposes of the treatment intervention and the expected outcomes, as this is likely to improve compliance with any negative consequences and gives a sense of control and decision-making to the patient. This can be aided by agreement on key words that represent the expected outcomes, e.g. a sense of freedom, embodiment, vitality. Involvement of the patient in the treatment process is likely to aid compliance and can be achieved in numerous ways. For example, when endeavouring to decide on a key component of the medicine, a choice could be given to the patient, perhaps giving them drop samples of different herbs and asking them to choose which they feel is the most suitable. Asking the patient if there are changes that they might make in their circumstances which would bring about improvement, to which the patient may suggest more exercise, taking up new pursuits, changes in diet etc. If these changes come from the patient they are more likely be to adhered to as many people are resistant to being told what to do.

The level of engagement of the medicine with the patient might be on a number of levels, for example, tissue or organ-based, concerned with physiological organisation or psycho-physiological balance or at a psycho-spiritual level. The choice of herbs or how they are applied determines the level of action.

For instance, the inclusion of a physiological astringent in a psychological combination has an action to tie the effect to the tissue level and preventing 'layering' of therapeutic effect, i.e. where the therapeutic effect works on an energetic level but doesn't connect with disharmony at the tissue and organ level and therefore is limited in extent.

The head and the body are interconnected, but it is easy to conceptualise them as separate. This is potentially problematic, as it could lead to the treatment of organs as separate from the systems that organise them, and hence not changing underlying aetiological factors. Functional change precedes organic change, i.e. it is relatively easy to change the dynamic equilibrium, but tissue change requires time.

Emotion

Emotion is important both in the sense that it is usually a major component in the aetiology of most illness and also as a general factor in terms of helping the movement of the intervention.

Unconditional positive regard is the default emotional framing for formulating medicines and for the consultation. Endogenous heat is an important principle in the therapeutic intervention. Physiologically it is representative of an inflammatory response, i.e. is an immunological process. Energetically it is linked to emotion, mainly anger and resentment. Where personal authority is compromised, a very common situation in childhood, by parents and other authority figures, the child becomes compliant but resentful—a pattern that often endures into adulthood. Anger and resentment are usually somatised, i.e. kept in the body and out of consciousness so they can be denied and not required to be acted upon. The process of releasing heat and emotion must be accompanied by a strengthening of personal authority and self-actualisation. Authentication is an important element to the consultation and medicine formulation. The importance of the feeling of the primal self of the patient makes it critical that the patient is always authenticated through the treatment intervention and that their fundamental worth and value are recognised and appreciated.

The unconscious only works well with authenticated experience, not ideas, and therefore the medicine should work on the affective domain of the patient. Where present, it is inevitable that heat and emotion are released during the intervention process and the medicine should be designed to aid resolution. It is not always necessary to discuss the nature and circumstances of historical abuse and trauma with the patient and, in fact, to do so may reignite the associated emotion and trauma. The resolution of negative emotional patterning is usually through a complex combination of factors, i.e. the building of personal resources in the patient, the authentication of the patient by the practitioner, the use of herbs to clear and resolve physiological conditions and the self-affirming choices and actions of the patient.

Illness as a behavioural construct

Illness is very much concerned with the situation of the primal self, which can have a strong vested interest in the condition and the circumstances surrounding it and hence be resistant to change. A strong motivation to change is therefore usually essential and needs to be established at the outset. The expectations, outcomes and consequences of the treatment need to be considered with the patient. As treatment progresses the patient becomes more aware of the implications of resolution, in terms of their psycho-social environment and circumstances, and may therefore become less compliant. The patient needs to have a clear idea of the benefits of resolution, feel that they have the resources to deal with the process and the outcome and feel as though this is a step forward. If this doesn't exist then a motivational goal needs to be put in place, e.g. a check list of all of the good outcomes that will occur following resolution. Sometimes the turning point for successful treatment is when the patient has reached rock bottom and makes a life-affirming choice of initiating change.

Sensorial impact

(See associated notes on tastes.)
The physical effects of the medicine, in terms of appearance and taste in particular, is very important and specific to the particular condition. For example, tonic medicines should taste and feel nourishing and supportive, medicines for treating infectious conditions should have a strong and reassuring taste, herbs for emotional support should be uplifting and supportive.

Care should be taken with bitter, astringent, and acidic herbs, by offsetting their taste with inclusion of suitable herbs, e.g. aromatics, demulcents, warming actions.

Qualities of herbs

- The temperature of a herb may be hot, cold, warming, cooling.
- The physical actions may be drying, moistening, astringing.
- The energetic actions may be nourishing, strengthening, transforming, harmonising, grounding.
- The direction of movement of the herb may be upward, downward, outward, inward.

Factors for prescribing

- Organ systems are interdependent and the function of a particular system is dependent upon the system as a whole.
- The overall constitutional state must be considered. What is the fundamental condition of the patient's vitality and essence?
- What is the direction of the illness? Is it compensatory, resolving or degenerative?
- Treatment should be supportive, but not compensatory or symptomatic.
- The body is in the control of the ANS. There is no distinction between the unconscious (instinctual, affective) and the body.
- The primary factor affecting the state of any organ is the functional balance, which is determined by the degree of constriction of the smooth muscle, i.e. state of congestion and energetic emphasis.
- Congestion promotes toxic build up and leads to organ depletion and vulnerability to invasion from infection and other pathogenic influences.
- Organ systems may be responding to exogenous or endogenous issues or circumstances.
- Treat causative factors rather than circumstances.
- Acute issues (acute symptoms) may have to be addressed before constitutional issues.
- The tissue state of the organ system is directly related to the functional balance and is affected by the efficacy of circulation nutritional status, pathogenic factors present and underlying constitutional state, all of which may have to be addressed to affect improvement.
- Acute conditions often need urgent and strong intervention, chronic conditions usually need cautious, less strong and persistent intervention.
- Dosage—start conservatively. Extreme deficiency requires low but sustained treatment. Rapid improvement is usually unsustainable. Care with the elderly.
- Tonification predisposes to action.
- Care is needed in conditions of extreme anxiety, overactivity, bipolar disorder.
- Medicines should 'inform' and lead to transformation.

Combinations of herbs

- Most herbs can be used together.
- Blood deficiency—priority for treatment. When nourishing the blood, include energy tonics, e.g. Angelica sinensis with Codonopsis.

- Combination of deficiency and major syndrome. Treat the syndrome first, particularly if serious. If the deficiency is considerable, treat both at the same time.
- Multiple organ deficiency—may need to prioritise. Digestive function is the most important because it is the foundation of the body requirement—nutrition. The adrenals are the second most important because they are the energy foundation.
- Assess the ANS, i.e. sympathetic deficiency or energy depletion?
- Energising herbs (sympathetic activators)—warm and dry. Care is needed with administration in situations of energy or blood deficiency because they consume energy. Need to include nourishing herbs.
- Nourishing herbs (parasympathetic)—cold, sweet and sometimes moist.
- Care is needed with administration in situations of congestion (damp, phlegm). May need to be balanced within the formula, e.g. add warm, aromatic herbs, e.g. citrus, Zingiberis.

There is no rule for the number of herbs included in a formulation. Herbs work well synergistically, and a sophisticated and efficacious effect can be achieved by combining herbal actions together. The whole is greater than the constituent parts. However, if the formulation is too complicated the patient may find it difficult to access or too confusing. Triads of herbs work particularly well, producing a stable and dynamic interaction. Triads can also be put together to form multiples or threes and this can also work very well.

Triads

Combinations of herbs can work extremely well together; with an augmentation and facilitation, which renders the combination greater than the sum of the parts.

Autonomy. Manifestation	Core energy. Foundational profile	Immune profile
Rosmarinus	Panax	Centella
Stachys	Schizandra	Astragalus
Verbena	Centella	Schizandra
Core resolution	**Liver heat syndrome**	**Kidney restorative**
Agrimonia	Arctium seed	Agropyron
Iris	Rosa	Alchemilla arvenesis
Carbenia	Althaea herba	Zea
Circulatory regulation	**Liver balance**	**Digestive regulation**
Achillea	Paeonia	Chamomilla
Crataegus	Iris	Potentilla
Leonorus	Bupleurum	Chicorium
Hormone regulation (pituitary)	**Menstrual regulation** (uterine)	**Oestrogen excess**
Salvia	Rubus	Paeonia
Aletris	Alchemilla vulgaris	Carbenia
Cimicifuga	Aletris	Glycyrrhiza

The herbal medicine formula

PRIMARY – The main and most important ingredient of the formula.
It treats the main syndrome, the main symptoms and the main cause of the illness.
It determines the principal function, character and application of the formula.
Usually a major tonic, adaptogen or balancing herb.

SECONDARY – Aids and enhances the actions of the primary herb.
One or more herbs may be used.
May be supplementary tonics to support the main ingredient, depuratives, nervines etc.

ADJUVANT – Used to deal with any additional or complicated signs and symptoms.
Also to moderate the actions of the main ingredients, e.g. astringent, bitter, ascendant, lymphatic, demulcent.

CIRCULATORY – Creates movement, usually upwards and outwards.
Controls the movement of the formula.

MESSENGER – Harmonises the whole formula. Assists the transport and movement of the herbs and prevents shock.
Synergistic, e.g. aromatic.

Dosages

When prescribing herbal medicines in material doses, the rules of pharmacy tend to apply, e.g. reduced quantity for the elderly, the frail, and children, and quantities are related to body mass and metabolism. Material doses may need to be delivered at particular times of the day to suit different organ systems. Generally lower doses are used for chronic conditions and larger doses for acute conditions.

Quantity is of less importance when prescribing energetically and the laws of pharmacy less relevant. Lower dosages tend to work more subtly and deeper, they are qualitative rather than quantitative and more impressionistic. A hint of lavender may work better on a state of anxiety or depression than a larger dose, but if you are using lavender to control a virus, and hence requiring a strong physiological action, then a strong medicine may be required. Energetic actions are more impressionistic and work on the 'feeling' dimension. Feeling is what ultimately determines physiological function.

Medicines should be given in dosages that optimise the balance of physical constituency, sensorial impact and appropriateness to the impact required. When treating acute conditions, or where support needs to be seen to be given, frequent administrations may be most effective, but for chronic conditions once or twice daily is usually sufficient and fits into the working day better. Dosages are not so relevant to the activity of the prescription but the same principle applies when treating the elderly, frail and children energetically, i.e. they are less able to tolerate vigorous interventions. Again, chronic conditions are generally treated slower and less vigorously than acute conditions.

There is often an assumption that there is a linear relationship between dose and outcome, i.e. small amounts of a medicine elicit small effects and large amount elicit large effects. This, however, is not always the case. We are intellectually shaped by pharmacy to consider that medicines with the same quantitative constituency will have consistently the same properties and actions. This is clearly not the case, even in pharmacy where individual responses to medicines can be inconsistent and unpredictable.

Hormesis

A term used in toxicology to represent a situation where positive outcomes follow a low exposure to a toxin or stressor, whereas large doses produce an inhibition. The response to dosage therefore follows a J-shaped, or possibly an inverted U-shaped, response curve. The mechanisms by which hormesis works are not well understood, but it could be that a low dose of a potentially physiologically problematic substance elicits the repair mechanisms of the body, but a large dose overwhelms them. This could be a factor in response to some herbal medicines, especially those which are potentially very damaging at a large dose.

Arndt-Schulz rule or Schulz' law

This is a related concept, which is now somewhat outdated. The Arndt-Schultz law states that weak stimuli increase physiological activity, whereas strong stimuli abolish or inhibit it. An extension of this law is called the type-effect hypothesis. The German physician Karl Koetschau described how the same substance at a small dose stimulates, a moderate dose stimulates and inhibits, and a large dose gives a short-lived stimulation followed by a strongly depressive effect. The net result is a stimulus followed by the response of the living system.

> The stimulus consists of the substance itself whose properties cannot be considered apart from the response. We can say, however, that according to this law of dosage a single substance can have different, often opposite properties at different dosage. Therefore, a single substance has no stable unchanging, predictable qualities.
> (Kenner & Requena, 1996, p. 256)

> There is further evidence, as we see later, that many herbs do not have properties that exist in any meaningful way outside the context of their field of activity, qualitatively or quantitatively. Quantitatively the dosage must be matched the to the vital capacity of the organism's immune response. Qualitatively, the activity of a substance is modulated by the nature of the terrain, the chemical make-up of the individual according to his constitutional type and living habits. The terrain is a concept in which biological individuality is the fundamental law, rather than an exception to the rule.
> (Kenner & Requena, 1996, p. 257)

Formulae for treating children

$$\frac{\text{Dilling: age in years}}{20} = \text{proportion of adult dose}$$

$$\frac{\text{Young: age in years}}{\text{Age in years}+12} = \text{proportion of adult dose}$$

Unexpected outcomes and defence reactions

- No perceived change by the patient. It happens! However, check the vital signs as patients soon move on and forget their symptom history.
- Acute symptoms. May be eliminatory, e.g. sickness and diarrhoea, colds, coughs and mucus. May be the re-emergence of previous acute symptoms, i.e. acute symptoms denote worsening or improvement as they are a vital response. The same with psychological symptoms; apathy, resignation and depression; are chronic, non-coping mechanisms.
- Shock/resistance. The patient may feel disturbed or experience the symptoms of internalised fear and it is indicative that there is difficulty coping with the promotional dynamic of the medicine, i.e. existential insecurity or releasing emotional blockages. Symptoms commonly are those of sympathetic deficiency/parasympathetic excess, i.e. muzzy-headed, tired, aching muscles, stiff neck, disturbed digestion, anxiety and/or depression, disturbed sleep. Resolve by 'grounding' the medicine, giving reassurance, taking things slower.
- The development of new symptoms, e.g. skin reactions, colds, phlegm, headache (cerebral resolution), joints. Follows the 'Law of Cure'. Problematic if it denotes a deepening pattern, i.e. new symptoms should be more externalised.
- Emotional reaction. Anger may lead to confrontation with the nearest, authority figures or the practitioner! Crying and distraught behaviour are common. Be supportive but don't reinforce negative reactions or suppress expression. It is a completely normal, acceptable and beneficial reaction.
- Transference and cross-transference. Can be therapeutically useful. Practitioners need to take care.

Contemporary actions of herbs related to traditional use

Contemporary action	Physiomedical action	Intervention	Examples of herbs
Diffusive Creates an outward and upward movement of blood and energy.	Diaphoretic. Relaxant and stimulant action on blood vessels. Encourages peripheral circulation in fever management, cardiovascular disease.	Engenders a sense of freedom and liberation. Maintains a sense of boundaries, integration and control. Leads to the release of conditions featured by fear, over regulation and control.	Achillea millefolium. Angelica archangelica. Anemone pulsatilla.

(Continued)

Contemporary actions of herbs related to traditional use (Continued)

Contemporary action	Physiomedical action	Intervention	Examples of herbs
Harmonising An action that unites functions together and integrates action throughout the nervous system. Action is centred in the head.	Relates to herbs that regulate and balance the autonomic and central nervous systems and which promote normal function of the neuro-endocrine systems. Stimulating and relaxing.	Creates a 'sense' of balance and integrity. Promotes the feeling of being in control.	Rosmarinus officinalis. Hyssopus officinalis. Hypericum perforatum.
Stabilising An action that creates tone (balance between stimulation and contraction) in the visceral organs. Action is centred in the body.	Relates to herbs that have a regulating action on the central metabolism, and includes astringents and many herbs that work on the liver, pancreas and digestive tract.	Creates a 'grounding' action. Promotes the feeling of having personal authority.	Agrimonia eupatorium. Carbenia benedictus.
Resolving Removes negative impression by a process of transformation. Involves a change in the emotional valency attached to important life events.	Depurative or cleansing herbs concerned with the removal of toxicity and combined with herbs with an aromatic quality. An extension of physical cleansing action to that of energetic cleansing action, i.e. the 'impression' which is associated with toxicity.	Removes complexes or internalised and unresolved emotional issues giving a sense of resolution and peace.	Paeonia laterifolia. Schizandra chinensis. Citrus aurantium flores.
Restoring An action which is positive and uplifting and which is counteractive to negative feelings and emotions.	Relates to herbs with a reputation as tonics or having nutritive benefit to the vital organs and tissues. The physically nutritional benefit relates to a sense of being nurtured.	Engenders a 'sense' of being nourished, loved, supported and respected.	Centella asiatica. Panax ginseng.

Herbs contraindicated in pregnancy

Care should be taken to avoid problematical herbs in prescriptions for women of childbearing age who could possibly become pregnant, particularly as herbal treatment can significantly improve fertility even when it is not the intended outcome. This is especially the case with herbs with potential cytotoxic effects as damage may be caused before pregnancy is confirmed.

In general, herbal medicine is not prescribed for the first trimester except for specific reasons. Herbs with the following actions or constituents are contraindicated:

- Emmenagogues
- Smooth muscle relaxants/stimulants
- Anthraquinones, alkaloids, essential oils
- Cytotoxic effects

Specific herbs contraindicated:

- Achillea millefolium
- Apium graveolens
- Artemisia spp.
- Berberis vulgaris
- Caulophyllum thalictroides
- Chelidonium majus
- Cimicifuga racemosa
- Cinnamon
- Cinchona spp.
- Crocus sativa
- Gossypium herbaceum
- Hydrastis canadensis
- Juniperis communis
- Magnolia lilifolium
- Mentha pulegium
- Oreganum vulgare
- Phytolacca decandra
- Rosmarinus officinalis
- Ruta graveolens
- Salvia spp.
- Sanguisorba canadensis
- Tanacetum vulgare
- Thuja occidentalis
- Thymus officinalis
- Viscum alba

This list is not exhaustive and the fact that a herb is not on it does not indicate that it is safe. In reality, the situation is much more complex as clearly safety has everything to do with dosage and the circumstances and constitution of the patient.

The qualities of flavour

	Sour	*Bitter*	*Sweet*
Movement	Cutting. Dispersing.	Dispersing. Downward.	Reassuring. Balancing.
Action	Stimulating. Carminative. Cooling.	Cooling. Detoxifying. Promotes digestion, stomach acid and assimilation. Stimulates bile. Antiviral.	Tonic. Demulcent. Nutritive. Nervine. Antispasmodic.
Excess	Acidity.	Cold.	Toxic. Damages the kidneys. Causes anxiety and tension.
Related organs	Liver—reduces excess activity. Tonifies the lungs. Anti-infective.	Heart. Tonifies the kidneys, but is depleting in excess.	Spleen-pancreas.
Complement	Reduces thirst. Moderated by pungent.	Counteracts sweetness, i.e. excess in the spleen. Balanced by salt.	Reduces pungency.
Constituents	H+, acids, ascorbic acid.	Alkaloids, bitter principals. Phenols, vol. oils.	Carbohydrates esp. sugars.
Examples	Sour foods; vinegar, acid fruit, tomatoes, wine, pickles.	Bitter vegetables (chicory, dandelion leaf) Angostora bitters.	Honey, dried fruits, grains.
Herbs	Schizandra, Citrus peel.	Gentiana, Rumex, Artemisia spp.	Panax, Althaea, Glycyrrhiza, Rehmannia.

Pungent	Salty	Aromatic	Hot	Cold
Disperses and releasing.	Moistens and softens.	Reassuring lifting.	Stimulating.	Sedating.
Stimulating. Diaphoretic, Carminative. Expectorant. Digestive. Warming. Stimulates body fluids.	Sedative, appetite stimulant. Demulcent. Aids circulation.	Raises energy and mood. Reassuring. Dispels shock.	Raises energy. Hypertrophic.	Decreases energy. Hypotrophic.
Burning—irritant and exhausting.	Looseness. Excess causes water retention, high blood pressure.	Nausea.	Burning. Drying. Excess.	Constriction. Deficiency.
Lungs, intestines.	Kidneys, adrenals and bladder.	Mind.		
Aids the digestion of sweet.	Aids sweet and excess balanced by sweet.		Cold.	Heat.
Alcohols, phenols, volatile oils.	Salts, minerals.	Volatile oils.		
Spices, onion and garlic family, chillies, cabbage family.	Sea salt, sea vegetables, celery, tamari.		Hot foods. Mustard. Chilli.	Cold foods. Salads.
Curcuma, Zingiberis, Armoracia.	Apium, Chodrus, Fucus.	Citrus flower. Hyssopus.	Capsicum. Zingiber.	

Tonics and adaptogens

> Inward calm cannot be maintained unless physical strength is constantly and intelligently replenished.
>
> (Buddha)

Fatigue relates to the fundamental or foundational energy status and depletion of the endocrine system, especially to adrenal function. Cortisol effectiveness may become deficient due to overstimulation of the stress response leading to either deficient production or cortisol resistance. The relationship to other hormone systems and to the neuroendocrine systems is intricate and complex. The relationship of the endocrine system to the autonomic nervous systems is also complex and intricate. Deficiency conditions and their effects on the hypothalamic and pituitary control pathways lead to impairment in function of the endocrine system, although sympathetic activation may occur as a compensatory outcome, i.e. fatigue may manifest as a deficiency or excess condition depending upon the circumstances. An individual may have an excess pattern when they are working due to a compensatory adrenergic response, but a deficient pattern when at rest, but both are due to the circumstances of fatigue. In fatigue the body will endeavour to reduce sympathetic output whenever circumstance permits, e.g. when at rest in the evenings and at weekends.

Fatigue syndromes can be related to the life events and lifestyle of the individual, e.g. excessive periods of stress, worry, exertion, overwork, death or separation from friends and relatives. These could be related to self-abusive regimes driven by negative emotion, such as guilt, burden of responsibility, lack of self-worth etc. and which are justified by social approbation. Recovery often requires a change in self-limiting beliefs and changes in life management and circumstances.

A deficiency pattern may relate to boundary problems and the sense of personal authority. There may be circumstances in which the individual feels restricted or disempowered and unable or incapable of taking remedial action, e.g. an abusive relationship, caring for a relative etc. Action on the part of the individual, to take control and change their circumstances, can be both a physical and mental liberation and change a fundamental feeling of self-worth. Authority may not be correctly engendered in the child, through the effects of parental manipulation, due to poor role modelling and the lack of engendering an archetype of the capacity to make decisions freely and effectively. To act in one's own best interest is to affirm self. Power is said to come from authority and authority comes from certainty.

Fatigue may accompany an improvement in the individual's circumstances, i.e. a post-traumatic reaction, e.g. retirement from a demanding job. A sustained period of high intensity work, often stressful and emotionally charged, can lead to fatigue factors that only become apparent when the circumstances change.

The immunological response of the body follows implicitly the balance of the ANS, behavioural reactions and physiological status, and infection both acute and chronic is frequently an important element in aetiology and in deterioration and chronicity, e.g. glandular fever. Many symptoms that are apparently indicative of infection are in fact fatigue induced, e.g. hot/cold, flu like symptoms, sore throat, glandular congestion. Congestion leads to the accumulation of toxic heat.

Depletion of energy, vitality or essence leads to feelings of inadequacy, vulnerability and anxiety, i.e. anxiety and depression may be consequent rather than causative and respond to tonics rather than sedatives. Fatigue may therefore present as anxiety and depression but the cause is in reality an underlying deficiency condition from fatigue. Common presentations of fatigue are a sense of fragmentation, overwhelm, inability to cope, disintegration. Depletion is often accompanied by a feeling of instability, which can be related to the traditional Chinese medicine concept of 'Wind'. The individual needs 'grounding'. Participation in mind-expanding activities or pursuits is contraindicated.

Adrenal fatigue

Terminology

Adrenal insufficiency. A medical condition referring to adrenal failure. May be primary adrenal deficiency or Addison's disease or secondary adrenal deficiency due to reduced ACTH secretion from the pituitary. Secondary is much more common. Adrenal insufficiency can progress to adrenal crisis: a serious and life threatening condition and a medical emergency. Addison's is in the majority of cases regarded as an autoimmune disorder, other causes are TB, trauma and malignancy (Betterle & Morlin, 2011).

Adrenal fatigue or hypoadrenia. A condition of varying degrees of deficit. It is a significant contributing factor in a wide range of medical conditions as well a major cause of problems with energy and well-being. Conversely, many conditions and their medical treatment can predispose towards adrenal depletion. Chronic fatigue syndrome is largely an adrenal fatigue problem, but in all cases of endocrine deficiency it is difficult separate different hormonal deficiency states. Adrenal fatigue is inevitably an endocrine deficiency problem and also linked to sex hormone, thyroid and growth hormone deficiency. Neurasthenia is a condition of fatigue, anxiety, lassitude, depressed mood, headache and neuralgia, which involves nervous system deficiency and compromised trophic condition of the tissue state, as well as adrenal fatigue. Adrenal fatigue typically affects the urinary kidneys and is a primary causative factor in CKD (chronic kidney disease).

Conditions with a strong association with adrenal fatigue:

- Arthritis
- Chronic fatigue syndrome
- Depression and anxiety
- Fibromyalgia
- IBS or chronic digestive problems
- Allergies
- Hypotension
- Hypothyroidism
- Hyperthyroidism
- Premature menopause
- Chronic anxiety
- Rage attacks
- Insomnia

Adrenal fatigue is the major element in deficiency conditions, i.e. passive sympathetic deficiency, where fatigue is connected with significant changes in mood, anxiety and depression, and sleep disturbances. Such conditions could easily be diagnosed as problems with mental health and treated accordingly, potentially leading to significant worsening of the condition.

Key signs and symptoms

Fatigue

Can manifest in a number of ways: generally feeling tired and rundown, difficulty getting up in the morning or feeling tired until late in the day, poor recovery from exertion, e.g. following a day of physical work, still feeling tired the next day. Sometimes unable to stop but exhausted when does so. Often feels more energy in the evening than during the day.

Muscular aches and pains

Muscle ache, especially in the lower back and knees, due to weakness in the supporting muscles rather than structural defect. 'Empty' neck and shoulders. Adrenal 'ache'. A deep, tender, ache in the back in the region of the kidneys.

Overwhelmed

Feeling overwhelmed by day to day events. Finding stressful situations unusually problematical or taxing. Feeling of 'fragmentation'. Vulnerability. Inexplicable anxiety.

Emotion/thinking patterns

Irritable. Anxiety attacks. Low mood. Pensiveness. Difficulty reframing ones thinking. Muzzy-headedness with poor mental focus and difficulty concentrating. Pessimism, hopelessness and despair.

Circulation

High or low blood pressure. Light headedness, instability, muzzy-headed and orthostatic hypotension.

Sleep

Can be excessive need to sleep or difficulty settling and waking up.

Hormones/libido

Low libido in men and women. Disturbed menstrual cycle and PMS in women. Loss of pubic hair and loss of body and leg hair.

Digestive disturbances

Abnormal weight gain, especially in the torso and thighs. Visceroptosis. Craving for salty and sugary foods and carbohydrates. Digestive disturbance, such as nausea, bloating, diarrhoea. Hypoglycaemia. Need for caffeinated drinks to 'get going'. Avoidance of foods with high potassium content, e.g. bananas, figs.

Chronic sodium-potassium imbalance

Low aldosterone leads to increased sodium excretion by the kidneys and net sodium deficiency and dehydration. This manifests as a craving for salty foods.

Temperature

Sweating, sensitivity to heat, excess sweating with exercise. Cold periphery.

Other indications of adrenal fatigue

Oversensitivity to noise and light. Hollow cheeks, i.e. a gauntness from loss of muscular tone.

Diagnostic characteristics of Addison's

Exacerbations of deficiency symptoms, e.g. malaise, anorexia, loss of libido, depression. Clinical signs include pigmentation (copper colouration, especially of the palmer creases from ACTH hypersecretion), vitiligo, weight loss, wasting, loss of body hair, hypotension. In general, indications of a reduction in sympathetic tone. Usually accompanied by disturbances of electrolytes and kidney function.

Orthostatic hypotension test

The patient lies down for approximately five minutes. After taking their blood pressure, stand the patient up and take the blood pressure again.

Increase of systolic blood pressure

Increases 6–10 mm/Hg	– Healthy adrenal function
No change	– Fair adrenal function
Drops 1–10 mm/Hg	– Poor adrenal function
Drops more than 10 mm/Hg	– Adrenal exhaustion

Difficulty in maintaining systolic blood pressure is due to poor epinephrine secretion and hence adrenal-medullary deficiency.

Paradoxical pupillary reflex

Adrenal fatigue is one reason for a shortened pupillary reflex.

Constriction for at least 20 seconds	– Normal function
Pulses after 10 seconds	
Pulses after 5–10 seconds	– Poor adrenal function
Immediate pulsation and dilation	– Adrenal exhaustion

Emotional response

Every emotional response has a behavioural component, an autonomic component and a hormonal component. The hormonal component includes the release of epinephrine, an adrenal-medullary response that occurs in response to stress and that is controlled by the sympathetic nervous system. The major emotion studied in relation to epinephrine is fear.

Treatment strategies for chronic fatigue and energy depletion

Sleep

One of the main purposes of sleep is for the recovery of the endocrine system. Good amounts of quality sleep are essential. Most authorities recommend going to bed no later than 10:30 pm and preferably allowing one's self to wake naturally in the morning. Sleep in the dark is also essential for melatonin production.

Exercise

Gentle exercise is vitality promoting but should fall considerably short of creating tiredness, which is counterproductive. Exercise should not be goal directed, i.e. it should be of a relaxed and enjoyable nature. Examples are walking in the woods, swimming, cycling, dancing. Hard exercise induces the stress response and leads to fatigue.

Diet

Eliminate white sugar in all its forms and caffeinated drinks. Reduce salt, but when used replace with sea salt. Reduce the dependency on refined carbohydrates and grains; the diet should focus on organic meat and fish, organic and biodynamic vegetables and fruit, organic free range eggs and a variety of nuts, seeds and pulses. Vitamin D is critically important.

Nutrient	Application	Dosages
Vitamin C with bioflavonoids (ratio 2:1)	Essential for the adrenal hormone cascade and as an antioxidant. Requirement increases with increased cortisol production.	Daily amounts dependent upon the individual. Requirement increased by the more chronic and severe the depletion. Typically 2,000–4,000 mg. NB: this is greater than can be achieved through diet alone.
Vitamin E (As mixed tocopherols high in β-tocopherol)	Not essential for the adrenal hormone cascade but important for antioxidant actions to sequester the free radicals produced in manufacture.	800 i.u. vitamin E (mixed tocopherols) daily.
Pantothenic acid	Converts into acetyl CoA, essential for the mitochondrial energy conversion, which is particularly high in cells concerned with adrenal hormone production.	1,500 mg daily.
Vitamin B6	A co-factor in a number of enzymatic pathways in the adrenal hormone cascade.	50–100 mg daily.
B Complex	The complete B complex is required in small amounts for the adrenal hormone cascade.	Should be naturally sourced and represent the required proportions, i.e. B6: 50–100 mg B3: 75–125 mg B12: 200–400 mcg.

(Continued)

Nutrient	Application	Dosages
Magnesium	Essential for cellular energy production especially for the cells concerned with the adrenal hormone cascade	400 mg Magnesium citrate needs vitamin C and pantothenic acid as co-factors. Best absorbed in the evening.

(Wilson, 2001)

Psychological

Self-limiting mindsets need to be resolved. A capacity for effective personal decision-making is essential, as well as good boundaries. Tonification leads to action. Fatigue is intrinsically linked to psychological factors. Overwork is sometimes unavoidable but can be activity engaged in as displacement or as an avoidance strategy. Resources include flexibility, adaptability, acceptance, openness, esteem, forgiveness.

Cellular metabolism

Mitochondrial DNA is the fundamental source of energy production involving the Krebs cycle. It is damaged by:

- Processed foods with high sugar, carbohydrates and unhealthy fats that produce free radicals
- Eating late in the day, when energy demands of the body are low
- High iron levels
- Inactivity—creates low energy demands on the cells
- Toxins from air, food, water etc.
- Radiation and electromotive forces

Solutions

- Low carbohydrate diet
- Exercise—increases energy demand
- Removal of free radicals
- Specialist herbs to aid regeneration, e.g. Lapacho.

Classification of herbal actions

Herbs that increase the tone of the body tissues. To assist oxygen-bearing elements in the blood, augmenting metabolic processes and promoting nutrition. They impart added strength and vitality.

(Bartram, 1995)

Tonics

Tonic medicines have the following features:

- Balancing, regulating, adaptogenic actions on the ANS system, which encompass physiological, emotional and psychological domains.
- General health benefits and promote longevity.
- Act to strengthen the fundamental reserves of the body particularly that associated with the adrenals.
- Restoring and nutritional qualities.
- No negative effects.
- Feel good to take and have a pleasant taste.
- A structural profile that informs the energetic profile.

> In the presence of abundant Yin, Yang is endless.
>
> (Chinese proverb)

The active expression of energy requires resources and can only be maintained when the resources are available. This includes the potential of the organs of the endocrine system and the nutritional substances needed to support them. Tonification should be moderated according to the fundamental state of depletion, an individual may be too weak to generate a response and could lead to deeper problems. Tonification may also need to be moderated in relation to the season. Strong tonification is usually inappropriate in the autumn and winter, when the energy dynamics are often waning, but may be appropriate in the spring and summer when the energy dynamics are rising.

Tonics are contraindicated in cases of acute infection and aggressively active cancer.

Regulating tonics Balance the CNS and ANS working upon the hypothalamic-pituitary regulation as well as directly upon the endocrine glands	Panax ginseng. Eleutherococcus sentinosus. Astragalus membraneous. Centella asiatica. Smilax officinale. Withania.
Nourishing tonics	Borago officinale. Symphytum officinale. Rehmannia glutinosa. Polygonum mutiflorum. Schizandra chinensis. Lycium, Glycyrrhiza glabra. Ligusticum porter. Asparagus, Fucus.
Cerebral-spinal tonics, relaxants and restoratives	Turnera diffusa.Tribulus, Panax, Chamaelerium luteum, Aletris farinose.Caulophyllum, Schizandra chinensis. Stachys betonica.
Tonics for the generative system	Panax ginseng. Turnera diffusa. Smilax officinalis. Serenoa repens. Withania.
Cellular tonics Facilitation of ATP	Lapacho. Astragalus. Curcuma. Anti-oxidants. Trace minerals. B vitamins. Co-enzyme Q10.

Blood tonification

In terms of the use of tinctures in 'energetic' application the concern is with the process of blood production, not the supply of nutrients as such. Iron deficiency is best dealt with by supplementation, dietary manipulation or specialist formulations.

Blood production depends upon the following factors:

- Energetic state—the production of blood is affected by deficiency and facilitated with the use of stimulants and central tonics, e.g. Angelica sinensis, Panax, Codonopsis, Eleutherococcus, Hydrocotyl, Rehmannia, Lycium, Echinacea.
- The absorption of iron is related to the qualitative tissue state of the membranes, i.e. congested; catarrhal membranes lead to inhibition of absorption. Absorption is facilitated by astringents and bitters, e.g. Agrimonia, Gentiana. Liver herbs are useful.
- The absorption of iron requires co-factors.
- Specific herbs for iron content and a physiological level, e.g. Rumex, Urtica.

Tonic formulations

1. Tonic herbs can be used together.
2. Energising herbs (sympathetic activators)—warm and dry. Care is needed with administration in situations of energy or blood deficiency because they consume energy. Need to include nourishing herbs.
3. Nourishing herbs (parasympathetic)—cold, sweet and sometimes moist. Care is needed with administration in situations of congestion (damp, phlegm). May need to be balanced within the formula, e.g. add warm, aromatic herb, Citrus, Zingiberis etc.
4. Combination of deficiency and major syndrome. Treat the syndrome first, particularly if serious. If the deficiency is considerable treat both at the same time.
5. Acute conditions often need urgent and strong intervention, chronic conditions usually need cautious, less strong and persistent intervention.
6. Blood deficiency—priority for treatment. When nourishing the blood, should include energy tonics, e.g. Angelica sinensis with Codonopsis.
7. Assess the ANS, i.e. sympathetic deficiency or energy depletion?
8. Multiple organ deficiency—may need to prioritise. Digestive function is the most important because it is the foundation of the body requirement—nutrition. The adrenals are the second most important because they are the energy foundation.
9. Dosage—start conservatively. Extreme deficiency requires low but sustained treatment. Rapid improvement is usually unsustainable. Take care with the elderly.
10. Combine with dietary advice. Avoidance of cold, greasy and indigestible foods and raw grains.
11. Tonification predisposes to action.
12. Care is needed in conditions of extreme anxiety, over activity, bipolar disorder.
13. Medicines should 'inform' and lead to transformation.

Herbs for tonification

Herb	Therapeutic movement	Principal therapeutic actions
Angelica sinensis	Warm. Pungent. Bitter. Sweet. Restorative, stimulating, relaxing.	Blood tonic. Antispasmodic. Ancillary Actions: Alterative. Hepatoprotective. Hormone regulator. Diuretic.
Astragalus membranaceus	Warm. Sweet. Aromatic.	Tonic. Immunostimulant. Adaptogen. Ancillary Actions: Hepatoprotective. Antibacterial, antiviral. Antioxidant. Hypotensive. Vasodilatory. Cardiotonic.
Atractylodes ovata	Sweet. Bitter. Nourishing. Warm.	Tonic. Diuretic.
Borago officinalis	Cold. Moist. Pungent and salty.	Adrenal tonic. Ancillary Actions: Depurative. Demulcent. Pectoral. Anti-inflammatory. Tonic. Antidepressant. Antispasmodic.

Conditions applicable and combinations	Energetic actions and notes
Female tonic to circulate and improve blood quality. Hormone regulator and oestrogenic stimulant for: Dysmenorrhoea. PMS. Menopausal symptoms. Infertility. Amenorrhoea. Depurative blood cleanser. Hepatitis. Liver restorative. Hypertension. Raynaud's disease. Atherosclerosis. Headache and migraine especially hormonally related. Strongly immune stimulating and anti-tumoural. **Special features: stimulating and relaxing, restorative and cleansing tonic for women in particular.** Maintenance of vitality and well-being.	Remedies for energetic clearing and protection. Balancing the 'heart'. Note differences from Angelica archangelica—root and herb. Angelica dahurica.
Acute and chronic viral infections. Immunostimulant and stimulant for leucocytosis. Interferone stimulant. Debility, fatigue, ME. Organ prolapse—uterus. Ischaemic heart disease. Hypertension. Palpitations. Excessive perspiration from deficiency. **Special features: vitality and energy tonic particularly for the immune system.** Tinnitus, blurred vision, dizziness from energy depletion.	In Chinese medicine is regarded as specific to tonifying the Wei Qi and more suitable for younger people.
Atractylodes is used as a general energy tonic and specifically a tonic for the digestive system and lungs. It is regarded in Chinese medicine as a regulator of the appetite and is used for weight regulation. It is also a diuretic used to regulate fluid metabolism.	
Adrenal weakness and dysfunction—specifically recovery from steroid therapy. Debility. Depression. Hepatitis. Jaundice.	Raises the spirits and emotions.

(Continued)

Herb	Therapeutic movement	Principal therapeutic actions
		Diaphoretic. Galactagogue.
Codonopsis pilusula	Sweet. Warm. Nutritive.	Tonic. Adaptogen.
Eleutherococcus senticosus	Warm. Moist. Sweet. Pungent. Stimulating, relaxing, restoring.	Tonic. Adaptogen. Ancillary Actions: Stimulant and sedative. Antispasmodic. Immunostimulant. Endocrine agent—aphrodisiac, gonadotrophic, adrenal tonic. Anti-inflammatory. Antiviral. Antifungal.
Eucommia ulmoides	Sweet. Warm.	Tonic. Anti-inflammatory.
Centella asiatica	Warm. Bitter. Astringent. Pungent. Stimulating. Relaxing, restoring.	Tonic. Adaptogen. Depurative. Stimulant and relaxant. ANS balancer. Bitter. Laxative. Diuretic. Anti-inflammatory. Antibacterial. Antifungal.

Conditions applicable and combinations	Energetic actions and notes
Membrane tonic and restorative—cystitis. Nephritis. Bronchitis. Rheumatoid arthritis. **Special features: tonic and restorative for debilitated conditions.** Raises sympathetic tone.	
Tonic and adaptogen. Codonopsis is regarded as essentially similar to Panax with the following differences: • It is milder and more appropriate where the hot, active energy of Panax may be overstimulating. • It is particularly useful for nourishing the blood and lungs, balancing the primary metabolic functions and for restoring hot, dry tissues states. • It is more suitable in conditions where there is 'false fire' symptoms, e.g. stiff neck and shoulders, headaches, high blood pressure, irritability etc.	Change of seasons soup— Codonopsis, Lycium, Astragalus, Dioscorea. Dragon Herbal— Codonopsis, Poria, Atractylodes, Glycyrrhiza.
Fatigue. Stress and anxiety. Depletion. ME. Blood sugar regulation—hypoglycaemia. Blood pressure regulation. Coronary and capillary circulatory tonic. Musculoskeletal circulatory deficiency. Rheumatism. Atherosclerosis. Cerebral circulatory insufficiency. Immune stimulation in chronic infection, candida, cancer. **Special features: tonic and adaptogen to improve vitality and energy.**	
Regenerative tonic for the liver and adrenals to enhance sympathetic energy and tone. Strengthens the bones, muscles, tendons and enhances healing of weakened and injured tissues. Particularly applicable to strengthen the lower back and for leg pain, stiffness and arthritis. Has considerable hypotensive action.	Bark use is not destructive to the tree. From the rubber family.
Fatigue. Anxiety. Depression. Insomnia. Impotence. Sexual dysfunction. Blood tonic and detoxifier for skin disorders, rheumatism. lupus, acne, sexually transmitted diseases.	Balances the ANS and CNS Balances right and left centres.

(Continued)

Herb	Therapeutic movement	Principal therapeutic actions
Ligusticum wallichiiw	Aromatic. Bitter. Warm and stimulating.	Trophorestorative. CNS stimulant. Astringent. Diuretic. Immunostimulant.
Lycium chinense	Sweet.	Tonic. Hepatic and hepatoprotective. Nephritic tonic. Antirheumatic.
Panax ginseng	Warm. Moist. Sweet. Pungent.	Tonic. Adaptogen. Ancillary Actions: Stimulant. Sedative. Thymoleptic. Endocrine agent—adrenal restorative, aphrodisiac. Antioxidant. Immunostimulant. Antineoplastic.

Conditions applicable and combinations	Energetic actions and notes
Leprosy. TB. Malaria. Tumours. Hepatic disorders. Hypercholesterolaemia. Cerebral circulatory stimulant and tonic—amnesia, memory, concentration difficulties. Strengthening of capillary and vein walls—varicose veins, haemorrhoids, microcirculation. Anticancer. **Special features: tonic and adaptogen for debilitating illness and tissue damage.** ANS balancer.	
Cerebral circulatory stimulant—dizziness, dementia. Gastrointestinal astringent—catarrhal and ulcerative conditions. Ulcerated conditions of all membranes—aphthous ulcers. Hypersensitivity and allergic reactions. Asthma. Menopause, metorrhagia. Hyperexcitability, irritability, insomnia. **Special features: tonic, stimulates blood circulation, particularly to the cerebral hemispheres and the eyes, and restores premature greying of the hair.** Hepatoprotective. Immunostimulant similar to Astragalus.	The Shen Nung says 'It is tonic to the vital centres, brightens the eye, strengthens the Yin, quiets the five viscera, nourishes the vital principal, makes vigorous the loins and navel, expels the hundred diseases, restores grey hair and if taken for a long time will increase the firmness of the flesh, giving sprightliness and youth to the body'.
Trophorestorative for the liver and kidneys and associated weakness of the eyes. Weakness in the legs and arthritis. Calming for the nervous system and heart. In Chinese medicine Lycium is regarded as a liver and blood tonic to increase vitality, brighten the eyes and improve night vision. Antioxidant and immune enhancing.	Prolonged consumption is said to promote cheerfulness.
Fatigue. Debility. Anxiety and depression. Insomnia. ME. Neurasthenia. ANS balancing. Pituitary regulator. To improve physical and mental endurance and stamina. Hypercholesteraemia. Hypoglycaemic.	In Chinese medicine used to strengthen the ancestral energy.

(Continued)

Herb	Therapeutic movement	Principal therapeutic actions
		Cardiotonic. Hypotensive. Corticosteroid type action.
Panax quinquifolium	Bitter. Sweet. Restoring, relaxing.	Tonic. Adaptogen. Nerve balancer and restorative.
Polygonum multiflorum Available as root or leaf	Bitter. Astringent.	Tonic. Nervine. Hepatic. Bitter. Laxative. Diuretic. Antispasmodic. Astringent. Anti-infective.
Poria cocos	Sweet.	Tonic. Diuretic. Anti-diarrhoeal. Sedative, antidepressant. Immune stimulant, antineoplastic.
Rehmannia glutinosa		Tonic. Adrenal trophorestorative. Anti-inflammatory. Antihaemorrhagic. Antipyretic. Laxative. Anti-inflammatory. Antihaemorrhagic. Antipyretic. Laxative.

Conditions applicable and combinations	Energetic actions and notes
Hepatoprotective. Cerebral circulatory tonic—to improve memory, concentration. Impotence, infertility, sexual dysfunction. Heart failure. Palpitations. **Special features: stimulating and relaxing tonic and adaptogen for debilitated conditions.**	
Similar to Panax with adaptogenic, strengthening action but is more relaxing and restorative. **Specific features: adaptogenic and immune restorative for stress induced damage.** For sensitive and burdened constitutions.	Balances and restores the higher autonomic centres. One of the best balancing and restorative tonics.
Exhaustion and debility. Neurasthenia. Infertility. Lack of libido. Pain and weakness in the lower back, knees and tendons. **Special features: a stimulating and relaxing substrate tonic for the adrenals, liver and pancreas particularly where there is nerve debility.** Premature greying of the hair.	Superb tonic specifically to underpin the nervous system. Safe and non-toxic for use in material doses. Used as an anti-ageing herb.
Diarrhoea. Acidity. A relaxing and tranquillising tonic for the nervous system and circulation. In Chinese medicine Poria is regarded as strengthening for the spleen and the general metabolic functions, tonifying to the blood and soothing to the heart and lungs. It is a Yin tonic, used to complement the Yang tonics, and is used in many formulae as an adjunct in the same way that Glycyrrhiza is used. It is a diuretic, which is regarded as strengthening to the bladder and kidneys and regulates the fluid metabolism.	
Tonic for the adrenals and liver. Immunostimulating. Hormone regulating—menopause. To aid the production and circulation of blood. Rheumatoid arthritis. **Special features: nourishing tonic for debilitated conditions particularly.** Associated with hormone deficiency. Hot and dry tissues and membranes, e.g. menopause.	Available raw and prepared, raw is better for heat and the prepared as a tonic.

(Continued)

Herb	Therapeutic movement	Principal therapeutic actions
Rhodiola rosea		Adaptogenic tonic. Stimulant. Hepatic restorative. Sexual stimulant. Nerve tonic, anti-fatigue, antidepressant, tranquiliser. Antineoplastic.
Rosmarinus officinalis	Stimulating, relaxing, restorative, resolving. Bitter. Pungent.	Digestive deficiency conditions. Headache from deficiency. Circulatory weakness. Adaptogenic. Antiseptic and immune enhancing.
Salvia officinalis	Cool. Dry. Bitter. Astringent. Pungent. Stimulating, restoring, circulating, resolving.	Tonic. Nervine restorative. Adrenal trophorestorative Astringent. Aromatic. Stimulant. Relaxant. Antispasmodic. ANS balancer. Antibioltic. Antifungal. Antiviral. Antiseptic. Anti-inflammatory. Hormone balancer.
Schizandra chinensis	Astringent. Sweet. Sour. Bitter. Salty. Restoring, circulating, stimulating.	Tonic. Antispasmodic.

Conditions applicable and combinations	Energetic actions and notes
Activating tonic—raises the sympathetic tone. Restorative for the endocrine and immune systems. Stimulates mitochondrial activity. Aids repair of DNA and chromosomal damage. For fatigue and debility syndromes Improves cerebral circulation. Sexual impotence and dysfunction.	
Stimulant, relaxing and balancing tonic with an affinity for the digestive tract. Cerebral-spinal stimulant and restorative, adrenal tonic.	Principal ANS balancing herb.
Anxiety, depression. Debility and weakness. Bacterial, viral, fungal infection. Immunostimulating tonsillitis, laryngitis, pharyngitis, gingivitis. Hormone imbalance. Infertility. Improves cerebral circulation. Hyperhydrosis. Sexual dysfunction—hyper or hypo. Suppresses prolactin release. **Special features: tonic and balancing to the ANS and CNS.** Sympathetic restorative. Hot flushes and menopausal sweats and hormonal disturbances at menopause.	See also: Salvia triloba. Salvia sclarea. Salvia miltiorrhiza (Dan Shen).
Hepatitis. To restore and protect against hepatic damage. Liver detoxicant. Adaptogen for stress tolerance. Fatigue. Allergic reactions especially skin conditions. Insomnia. To improve cerebral circulation. Sexual dysfunction. Infertility night sweats. Blood heat conditions. Chronic coughing. Membrane dryness and irritability. Diarrhoea.	For the symptoms of false fire. To circulate the 'fire energy'. The five flavours.

(Continued)

Herb	Therapeutic movement	Principal therapeutic actions
Smilax off.	Warm. Moist. Pungent. Bitter. Sweet.	Tonic. Depurative. Hepatoprotective. Hormone stimulant and tonic. Immune stimulant. Anti-inflammatory. Diaphoretic.
Tabebuia spp. Lapacho Pau d'arco	Stimulating, restoring.	Immuno-stimulant. Antimicrobial. Antiparasitic, antifungal. Depurative. Anticancer. Anti-inflammatory.
Turnera diffusa	Stimulating, restoring. Bitter. Pungent.	CNS stimulant. Aphrodisiac. Nerve trophorestorative, thymoleptic. Diuretic Laxative.
Withania somnifera		Adaptogen. Nervine. Depurative. Anti-inflammatory. Antibacterial. Leucocytosis stimulant. Spasmolytic. Sedative.

| *Conditions applicable and combinations* | *Energetic actions and notes* |

GIT disturbance.
Special features: stimulating and relaxing tonic for energy strengthening and restoration particularly with nerve weakness and degeneration.

Blood and liver cleanser for chronic skin and joint diseases—psoriasis, gout, rheumatoid arthritis.
Mercurial poisoning.
Sexual dysfunction.
Impotence.
Infertility.
Catarrhal membranes Immune enhancer.
Endocrine and pituitary enhancer.
Itching skin conditions.
Special features: adrenal tonic and restorative—builds muscle weight and tone.
Blood purifier.
Anti-inflammatory.

Anticancer.
Chronic skin conditions, i.e. eczema, psoriasis, fungal infections.
Recovery and stability of cellular DNA.

Stimulant to the digestive tract—dyspepsia, constipation. Enuresis, irritable bladder
Prostatic hypertrophy.
Amenorrhoea, dysmenorrhoea.
Premature ejaculation and sexual weakness.
Special features: stimulating tonic, restorative and balancer for the CNS and ANS in depressed, debilitated and deficient conditions and with particular connection to the generative system.
Impotence, sexual deficiency and sexual dysfunction in both sexes.

Tonifies and balances the CNS, endocrine system and pulmonary/cardiac system. Improves cerebral function.
Impotence and sexual dysfunction.
Senile dementia.
Debility.
Special features: for chaotic, agitated, manic nerve patterns.
Can bring a sense of inhibition where this is not present.

English tonics and adaptogens

Tonic medicines have the following features:

- Balancing, regulating, adaptogenic actions on the ANS system, which encompass physiological, emotional and psychological domains
- General health benefits and promote longevity
- Restoring and nutritional qualities
- No negative effects
- Feel good to take and have a pleasant taste
- A structural profile that informs the energetic profile

e.g. Salvia. Hyssopus. Rosmarinus.

Herb	Actions	Uses and applications	Notes
Angelica archangelica Apiaceae Herba/radix Also: Angelica sinensis Andgelica dehurica **Key feature: Stimulating and relaxing tonic**	Warm. Dry. Bitter. Pungent. Sweet. Restoring, stimulating and relaxing. Antispasmodic, carminative. Antibacterial, antifungal, antiseptic. Bitter. Diuretic. Cholagogue.	Circulatory insufficiency. Vascular disease— Intermittent claudication. Headache and migraine. Respiratory infections, bronchitis, coughs, asthma. Dyspepsia. Appetite stimulant. Alcoholism. Menopausal symptoms. **Special features: a stimulating and relaxing diffusive tonic.**	Protective and opening. Emphasis on the head and higher centres. Caution: Pregnancy. Photosensitisation. Inflammation of the GIT.
Arctium lappa Asteraceae Constituents: Artiin—a bitter glycoside. Arctigenin— lignan. Inulin. Polyacetylines. Volatile oil. Terpenoids. Mucilage. Tannin. **Key feature: Adaptogenic alterative**	Bitter. Cooling. Aromatic. Sweet. Nourishing. Depurative. Tonic. Ancillary Actions: Hepatic, Cholagogue. Diuretic, antirheumatic. Diaphoretic. Lymphatic. Antiseptic, antibacterial, antifungal.	Elimination of toxins through the liver, kidneys and lymphatics—arthritis, sciatica, gout, eczema. psoriasis, acne, furunculosis and all skin and mucous membrane irritated conditions. Stimulating and restoring tonic for the liver and pancreas— hypoglycaemic,	Seed is particularly beneficial for the skin. Leaf for the GIT and as a diuretic Root for tonic properties.

(*Continued*)

Herb	Actions	Uses and applications	Notes
		antidiabetic, hepatoprotective. Antioxidant. Cystitis. Chronic glandular enlargement. Anti-tumour. Induces differentiation in tumours and inhibits proliferation in leukaemia. Regulates immune response and inhibits TNF production. Antimutagenic. **Special features: a powerful, stimulating and tonic depurative for all conditions of blood and lymph toxicity especially skin and rheumatic conditions.**	
Borago officinalis Boraginaceae Constituents: Alkaloids. Saponins. Mucilage. Tannins. Essential oil **Key feature: Adrenal Restorative**	Cold. Moist. Pungent. Salty. Adrenal tonic. Ancillary actions: Depurative. Demulcent. Pectoral. Anti-inflammatory. Tonic. Antidepressant. Antispasmodic. Diaphoretic. Galactagogue.	Adrenal weakness and dysfunction—specifically recovery from steroid therapy. Debility. Depression. Hepatitis. Jaundice. Membrane tonic and restorative—cystitis. Nephritis. Bronchitis. Rheumatoid arthritis. **Special features: tonic and restorative for debilitated conditions. Raises sympathetic tone; lifts the spirits and emotions.**	Lifts the spirits, calms and reassures.
Inula helenium Asteraceae **Key feature: Tonic pulmonary agent**	Bitter. Pungent. Warm. Restoring, stimulating, decongesting. Diaphoretic. Diuretic. Alterative.	Stimulating, warming and relaxing for fatigue, debility, immune deficiency with tendency to infections.	Potential as a major herb for the treatment of immunological deficiency and autoimmunity.

(Continued)

Herb	Actions	Uses and applications	Notes
		Chronic bronchitis, asthma, chronic parenchymal lung disorders. Infections of the lungs, bladder and urinary tract. Enhances immune potential. Toxic conditions such as eczema. Promotes oestrogen and progesterone insufficiency and hence menstrual deficiency. **Special features: stimulating, relaxing and warming pectoral tonic and immune enhancer.**	Has pituitary action, i.e. acts on the higher autonomic centres.
Rumex crispus Polygonaceea Constituents Volatile oil. Anthraquinone glycosides. Tannins. **Key feature: Blood tonic and alterative**	Cold, Dry. Bitter. Astringent. Decongesting. Restoring. Depurative. Ancillary Actions: Bitter. Hepatic, splenic, cholagogue. Antiseptic. antibacterial. Lymphatic stimulant. Laxative.	Blood tonic and cleanser Hepatic congestion, jaundice, cholagogue. Chronic membrane catarrh and irritation. Chronic skin conditions— eczema, psoriasis, prutritis, dry skin. Chronic inflammatory conditions. Breast congestion and lymphadenopathy. Constipation and mucous congestion. Aphthous ulcers, upper digestive ulceration. **Special features: stimulating depurative for the removal of conditions of toxic heat.** Stimulating tonic especially for improving blood quality.	Skin with guaiacum smilax. Similar in properties to Polygonum multiflorum.

(*Continued*)

Herb	Actions	Uses and applications	Notes
Symphytum officinale Boraginaceae Pyrrolizidine alkaloids Volatile oil **Key feature:** **Repair and regeneration**	Cool. Sweet. Moist. Softening. Hepatoprotective. Haemostatic (tannins). Demulcent. Vulnerary. Anti-inflammatory. CNS sedative (alkaloids). Nutritive.	Calms, restores and nourishes in dry deficient conditions. Demulcent. Anti-inflammatory. Vulnerary cell proliferant. Stimulates osteoblast and fibroblast activity. Nutritive.	Deep regenerative action on subtle as well as physical levels.
Taraxacum officinale Asteraceae **Key feature:** **Renewal**	Sweet. Moist. Resolving. Dissolving. Reassuring. Connecting.	Hepatic heat and congestion—eczema, acne, herpes. Restorative action for the liver, pancreas, adrenals, kidneys and connective tissues. Specific for deep muscular tension. **Special features: cleansing, harmonising and relaxing tonic and restorative for the liver, gall bladder, pancreas, GIT and kidneys for both deficiency and excess conditions.**	Releases deep patterns of emotional tension, especially associated with the liver. Establishes balance and reassurance.

Case history: fatigue

This 63-year-old lady complains of persistent fatigue, which has been worsening over a period of three years. She feels as though she has been through a life transition where many problematic events have happened, e.g. the death of her father, her husband's health problems, her sister developing cancer. She feels that she is no longer coping, feels fragile and has negative thought patterns. She is inclined to feel the cold and has cold peripheries. Her shoulders feel stiff and her muscles heavy.

Clinical signs:
Blood pressure: 120/80.
Pulse: 66.
Pulse pressure: 40.
CVI: 13,200.
Tongue: slight heat to the tip.

Herb	Dosage	Actions
Angelica sinensis	15.00	Blood tonic. Moving to the circulation. Spasmolytic.
Centella asiatica	20.00	CNS and ANS regulator. Tonic and adaptogen.
Panax ginseng	20.00	Tonic and adaptogen. Regulation of the endocrine system. Engenders strength and capability.
Schizandra chinensis	10.00	Adjunct to the tonics.
Agrimonia eupatorium	15.00	Astringent liver tonic. Resolves emotional tension and heat.
Glycyrrhiza glabra	20.00	Nourishing tonic and adaptogen.
Borago officinale	20.00	Adrenal tonic and restorative.
Verbena officinale	15.00	Nervine restorative.
Rosmarinus officinalis	15.00	ANS balancer.
Flower essences: Olive Cherry Plum Walnut Hornbeam Agrimonia	7 ggt aa	Acceptance. Trust. Adaptability to change. Restoration.
Dosage: 5 ml bid aq ac.	150.00	

Two weeks:
Blood pressure: 132/78.
Pulse: 74.

One week agitated. One week much improved.

Twelve weeks:
Blood pressure: 132/62.
Pulse: 70.
Tongue: colour normal, no heat to the tip.

Energy, well-being and vitality much improved.

Case history: deficiency from fatigue

The patient is a senior manager of a manufacturing company and aged 44. This man complains of persistent anxiety. The anxiety occurs daily and appears unrelated to his day to day activities and he has no particular ongoing concerns. He reports his family life to be normal and his work life to be busy and stressful but not overwhelming. The anxiety has been worsening over a period of about three years. He has also had two panic attacks in the last few months.

He suffers from chronic indigestion and daily episodes of bloating and turbulence, but with normal bowel movements. He follows a gluten-free diet, which significantly improves his digestion. He has frequent anorexia and can easily miss a meal without undue effect. He has rosacea, which disappears with the gluten-free diet.

His head feels 'cloudy', he has significant problems with his focus and concentration, and his short term memory is poor. He has a persistent daily headache above his left eye. He describes his energy as generally low and especially poor in the mornings upon waking and in the evenings. He is considerably tired on weekends and days off. His sleep is described as disturbed and not restful, he has intense dreams. He has significant night sweats. His temperature generally is described as normal. He describes his libido as poor. A systems research did not reveal any other issues.

He is of slim, athletic build, is well-groomed and dressed in a fashionable suit. He appears a little tense but is articulate and sociable.

Orthodox medicine: Citalopram 20 mg for 18 months (no observable effects).

Biomedical considerations:
An endoscopy and blood tests reveal no abnormalities. His health is assessed annually through an employer operated health screening.

Clinical signs:
Blood pressure: 116/78.
Pulse: 70.
Pulse pressure: 38.
Tongue: significant swelling, especially to the sides, pale and flabby, heat from papillae to the tip, rear phlegm coating. Significant central cracking.

Diet and lifestyle:
He follows a strict gluten-free diet with plenty of fruit and vegetables.
No dietary supplements.
Limited alcohol consumption. Alcohol containing gluten is very poorly tolerated but he is able to consume gin and vodka in moderate quantities.

Interpretation and analysis:
A discussion took place with the patient concerning the nature of his anxiety. He felt that there were not any particular discernible problems but more of a sense of being overwhelmed and 'fragmented'. These feelings are typical of someone who has been overworking and stressed for a long time and suggest the onset of a fatigue issue. He reported that he generally feels better when he is at work; this suggests that when working he is more sympathetically connected. His clinical signs suggest a sympathetic autonomic system deficiency, and his pulse pressure is 38 against an expected norm of 50; there is perhaps some degree of constraint, as suggested by the diastolic blood pressure reading and clearly the systolic is inadequate in its compensation. This would account for the symptoms of cerebral blood flow deficiency, i.e. 'foggy' headedness, poor memory, focus and concentration and headache. The sympathetic deficiency could be considered from two perspectives. A passive deficiency as a consequence of a fatigue syndrome, the

body invoking a deficiency pattern in an effort to conserve resources. This would very much relate to the morning and evening fatigue, and fatigue at weekends. The pale and swollen tongue with a central fissure would support this, Chinese medicine would normal consider a pale and swollen tongue in a man as due to kidney deficiency, or in Western terminology, adrenal cortical fatigue.

The fissure in the tongue would suggest that there is a movement of the fatigue syndrome into the organic or tissue level, a more serious and deeper problem. The other consideration is that the sympathetic deficiency is active in nature, i.e. is a psycho-physiological restraint against his perceived psycho-social interconnection or in other words his life is too full, too complicated or overburdened. In reality the active and passive deficiency considerations are probably inter-related, i.e. being overburdened and overworked is a prerequisite for the development of a fatigue syndrome and a fatigue syndrome engenders a sense of fragmentation, inability to cope and feeling overwhelmed. This would follow from the age of patient, by the age of 44 it is common for busy people to reach the exhaustion phase of Selye's General Adaptation Syndrome (Ogden, 2012). He would also be at the nadir of the 'U-shaped happiness curve'. This well documented finding suggests that people are at their happiest in their teens and 70s but at their lowest in the their 40s (Hawkes, 2012).

It is also possible that he has a 'sensitive' personality, i.e. someone who has a trait leading to a sensitive central nervous system, related to the deep processing of physical, social and emotional stimuli. A sensitive person could be considered to have problems with boundaries. The fissure in the tongue could be construed as a fragmentation of his sense of self and capacity to cope (Aron, 1999).

The relationship of the gluten sensitivity to the deficiency pattern and fatigue is complex. A deficiency pattern leads to an increase in visceral function and consequentially a likelihood of increased immune-mediated response to potential irritants and allergens. An immune response involves histamine release and other pro-inflammatory substances, which in turn require cortisol to moderate. Cortisol is the major regulator of inflammation. The more histamine that is released, the more cortisol it takes to control the inflammatory response and the harder the adrenals have to work to produce more cortisol. Chronic allergy is therefore likely to lead to cortisol deprivation or adrenal fatigue (Wilson, 2009). Adrenal fatigue leads to a deficiency state, which compounds the problem. Conversely, sensitivity or allergy creates inflammation that induces an internalisation of function. It could also be argued that a sensitive person with poor boundaries may have increased physiological vigilance and therefore a sensitised immune response (Stableford, 2017). Intense dreams are often associated with overactivity of visceral function and the associated heat and restlessness.

Therapeutic intervention:
The therapeutic intervention is designed to bring about a deep acting tonification which will not only work upon the endocrine system but also on his sense of personal integrity and strength. It is important that the medicine does not induce any unacceptable deconstruction or unachievable psychological goals, these may interfere with his capacity to process the actions of the medicine.

Key actions:
Resolution and transformation of the personal self and facilitating manifestation. Building foundation energy, adaptability and resilience.

Herb	Dosage	Actions
Panax ginseng	15.00	Foundation energy. Affirmation of the sense of self and personal power.
Schizandra chinensis	10.00	Movement of the 'fire' principal. Adjunct to tonification.
Agrimonia	10.00	Resolution and integration.
Borago officinalis	20.00	Adrenal tonification and the courage to move forward.
Stachys betonica	20.00	Cerebral circulatory tonic.
Verbena officinalis	15.00	Nerve restorative and activator.
Rosmarinus officinalis	15.00	ANS balancer. Becoming manifest.
Flower essences: Agrimony, Larch, Walnut, Cherry Plum	7 ggt aa	Agrimony: acceptance and resolution of inner conflict. Larch: confidence and belief in self. Walnut: free from unheeded influences. Cherry Plum: trust in the higher process, that all will work out fine.
Dosage: 5 ml bid aq ac.	105.00	

In the first Chinese Material Medica, written some 2,000 years ago, Shen Nung said of ginseng that:

> Ginseng is a tonic to the five viscera, quieting the animal spirits, stabilizing the soul, preventing fear, expelling the vicious energies, brightening the eye and improving vision, opening up the heart benefiting the understanding and if taken for some time will invigorate the body and prolong life.
>
> (Teeguarden, 1984, p. 78)

The key to the intervention is a restorative, nourishing and affirming action to the endocrine system. Panax and Schizandra are an integral combination aimed at sympathetic restoration, endocrine tonification and the associated 'sense of' balance and power. Panax and Schizandra, in particular, tonify the endocrine system and underpin the circulation, digestion system and nervous system (Hempton & Fischer, 2009). They note that Panax is contraindicated in situations of Yin deficiency, i.e. the nutritional requirements needed to underpin the building of energy must be in place.

Agrimonia has the bitter, astringent qualities to assist the elimination of endogenous heat together with the resolvent quality of the Rosa family, which helps with the resolution and integration of associated internalised emotional tensions (Stableford, 2017). Borago offers further support to adrenal cortical function and the associated facility of the courage to deal with one's situation (Mrudula et al., 2016).

The combination of Stachys, Verbena and Rosmarinus will have actions in terms of the physiological tonification and support of the nervous system, but at an energetic level will work together to become messengers to the autonomic control processes in the limbic brain—bringing a sense of connection to one's self and the world, enhancing sensorial experience and a feeling of personal integration. These herbs have an affinity for the head and one's sense of control and regulation. To be manifest is to feel alive and connected (Stableford, 2017). Rosmarinus, in addition to the autonomic regulating actions, is relaxing, stimulating and tonifying for the digestive system, optimising function.

Prognosis:
The patient will experience a stronger sense of self, the feeling that he is more in contact and 'alive' in the world, more allowing in letting good things happen for him, a stronger, more adaptable and resilient foundation energy. Change is expected to be steady over a period of perhaps six months.

Two weeks:
Blood pressure: 114/68.
Pulse pressure: 46.

Some improvement in energy. Experienced several days of turmoil but has felt better in mood since. Has experienced sleep of better quality and shorter duration.

Six weeks:
Blood pressure: 110/66.
Pulse: 64.
Pulse pressure: 44.

Improvement in energy and mood.

Ten weeks:
Blood pressure: 110/64.
Pulse: 66.
Pulse pressure: 46.

Energy improved. Head is clearer. Nocturnal sweating improved. Still some intense dreams. He has noticed a significant change in his communication with others, being more relaxed and open.

The decision was made to further develop the medicine. The psycho-social interconnection of the patient seems to have improved, but further work is needed on the fatigue syndrome and so additional tonics were added to the formulation, notably, Astragalus membraneous and Polygonum multiflorum.

Herb	Dosage
Panax ginseng	20.00
Astragalus membraneous	20.00
Schizandra chinensis	10.00
Agimonia	10.00
Polygonum multiflorum	20.00
Borago	20.00
Stachys	20.00
Verbena	15.00
Rosamirinus	15.00
Dosage: 5 ml bid aq add.	150.00

Fourteen weeks:
Blood pressure: 116/72.
Pulse pressure: 44.

A significant improvement in energy, well-being and mood. The night sweats have been absent.

The patient experienced significant digestive problems, following ingestion of gluten at a conference. The symptoms of the gluten reaction were not as pronounced, and the rosacea did not reoccur. The diastolic blood pressure may be raised due to liver sensitivity to immunological reactivity.

The nervous system

Classification of mental illness

The classification of mental illness can be problematical, as there can be a cultural and social perspective, different cultures have different norms and expectations. Classification is primarily to serve prescribing practice and serves little to provide an aetiological explanation of causes. Classification has a categorical sense to it, that it is somehow fixed and immutable, and therefore gives a mindset that change is problematical. There is generally a great deal of overlap between conditions.

Rosenhan and Seligman's seven features

- Suffering. Suffering is a normal part of life and is not necessarily indicative of abnormality and there are those with an abnormality, e.g. personality disorder, who do not appear to suffer themselves despite causing suffering in others.
- Maladaptiveness. Maladaptive behaviour is behaviour that prevents an individual from achieving major life goals, having fulfilling relationships with others or working effectively (for instance an agoraphobic will not venture out of the house due to fear).
- Vividness and unconventionality. Vivid and unconventional behaviour is relatively unusual. It is behaviour that differs substantially from the way that you would expect normal people to behave in similar situations. However, there are many people who behave in this way that are not deemed to be abnormal.
- Unpredictability and loss of control. With most people, you can normally predict what they will do in known situations. In contrast, abnormal behaviour is often highly unpredictable, uncontrolled and inappropriate for the situation.
- Irrationality and incomprehensibility. One of the characteristics of abnormal behaviour is that there appears to be no good reason why the person should choose to behave in that way.

- Observer discomfort. Our social behaviour is governed by a number of unspoken rules about behaviour, such as the way we maintain eye contact or personal space. When others break these rules we experience discomfort. But this does not necessarily indicate abnormal behaviour, for instance different cultures may well have different social rules about behaviour.
- Violation of moral and ideal standards. When moral standards are violated, this behaviour may be judged to be abnormal.

Traditional classification

Neurosis

Mild illness where the impairment can be seen and understood as an extension of normal behaviour. The individual generally has a perspective of their condition and reality in general.

- Anxiety
- Hypochondriasis
- Insomnia and sleep disturbances
- Hyperactivity
- Psychosexual disorders

Psychosis

Severe illness where the impairment is beyond what can be accepted as normal behaviour. Sometimes regarded as 'organic' in nature. Generally, involves a disturbance of the processing of reality.

- Schizophrenia: Type I—acute (delusions, hallucinations); Type II—flattened affect, communication difficulties
- Paranoia
- Clinical depression
- Bipolar—manic depression

Personality disorder

Personality disorders span a range of presentations, from that which is highly problematic to the individual and society, to that which would be considered to be part of everyday life.

- Psychopathy
- Sociopathy
- Subcultural deviance

Conditions where there may be significant pathophysiological presentations. Help may be given from the constitutional perspective but serious organic and intractable circumstances may pertain.

- Epilepsy
- Trigeminal neuralgia
- Neuritis

Degenerative brain disorders	Non-degenerative brain disorders
Alzheimer's	Vascular dementias, e.g. multi-infarct dementia
Extrapyramidal syndromes, e.g. progressive supernuclear palsy	Infectious dementia, e.g. AIDS dementia
	Neurosyphilis
Wilson's	Post-traumatic
Huntingdon's	Demyelinating disorders, e.g. multiple sclerosis
Parkinson's disease	Toxic and metabolic disorders, e.g. vitamin deficiencies B12, niacin
Frontotemporal dementia	
Cortico-basal dementia	Chronic alcohol or drug abuse, e.g. Korsakoff syndrome
Leukodystrophies, e.g. adrenoleukodystrophy	
Prion-related dementias, e.g. Creutzfeldt-Jakob disease	

(Kolb & Whishaw, 2003)

Anxiety

Anxiety is a feeling that informs of a problem with one's boundaries and that an external loss or intrusion has occurred combined with a low sense of confidence in being able to solve the problem. The intrusion can be on different levels, physical and psychological. Boundary problems are often reflected in expressions, such as overwhelmed, stressed, out of control. The formation of good boundaries is essential in the development of a strong sense of self, independent decision-making, integrity and authority. Poor boundaries engender a sense of vulnerability and dependency, which in turn can result in a sense of humiliation and anger. Boundaries define who we are and form our identity, preferences and beliefs. It is important to be able to define what is inside one's boundary and what is outside, and to identify when unwanted and unhelpful intrusions occur. In an ideal world, boundaries wouldn't be necessary, if one was completely clear and confident in one's self, but in most circumstances, boundaries need to be built and maintained and the nature of the boundary can be changed in relation to one's self-development. In many ways, the establishment of a firm boundary is a 'rite of passage', which requires courage and determination. The main step in the formation of a firm boundary is usually taken with one's parents, where they have to be made aware in definite terms that one is an independent individual with whom they can have a relationship with but whom they do not control. One's boundary is an inalienable right and without it one's resources are in danger and there is a limitation on one's self-emancipation.

The relationship between boundaries and resources is complicated and reciprocal. Poor resources, in terms of both psychological, e.g. low self-esteem and poor self-belief and physical, e.g. poor energy foundation and physical integrity, lead to a weakened sense of boundary, whereas good resources help towards the establishment of good boundaries through the development of strength and capability. Anxiety is therefore not usually so much to do with reassurance but in building the constitution to support a movement towards self-actualisation, otherwise there may be a development of dependency upon continued reassurance.

Anxiety may be the presenting symptom of a deficiency condition, such as passive sympathetic deficiency resulting from fatigue. This is a common presentation in middle and old age and it is important to distinguish the condition from psychological anxiety, as the use of relaxants and sedatives worsens the condition. Instead tonics are required to lift the sympathetic tone. Mood and sense of safety are dependent upon the profile of the autonomic nervous system.

Depression

Low mood may be a feature of an autonomic sympathetic deficiency, where internalisation of function inevitably results in low energy, poor sense of vitality and aliveness, introspection, lethargy and low mood. However, depression in its true form is a common reaction to hurt and is a mechanism to block feeling, usually of anger. Anger is the reaction to humiliation, where one's sense of personal authority is compromised. The main antidotes to depression are feeling, decision making and assertion. Well-being strengthens the protection against hurt.

Emotionality may be said to be on a continuum between anger and anxiety, i.e. anger(rage)–neutrality–anxiety(terror).

All emotional expression is a combination of both, e.g. irritability, a combination of some anger and some anxiety.

– Positive emotionality: self-esteem = well-being (feeling nurtured) + confidence (self-belief).
– Negative emotionality: anger and/or anxiety when self-esteem is compromised.

Well-being strengthens our protection against hurt. Depression is a common reaction to hurt as it blocks feeling. Making a decision is the best way out of depression. The negative reaction to hurt is to hurt back. Society deals with aggression by hurting back, which leads to a cycle of violence. Assertion is the antidote to anger as it demonstrates implicitly that one is no longer a victim and is in control (Dobransky, 1999).

Herbal actions

Trophorestoratives

Anxiety, tension, depression and insomnia may be both a cause and a consequence of debility within the nervous system tissue and is inseparable within the concept of curative treatment. 'Neurasthenia' refers to a debilitated tissue state of the nervous system. Herbal therapeutic principles recognise that anxiety, tension and depression are not only behavioural responses but are intrinsically linked with energy status and endocrine balance, and treatment may be more appropriately involved with nourishing, strengthening and hormone regulation than with simply making the patient comfortable. Tranquillity comes from strength. Assessment and treatment of all system pathways is indicated. Toning and balancing of the autonomic nervous system is inevitably appropriate. Nutritional status and diet need to be addressed. Herbs with stimulating, relaxing, balancing and restorative actions.

Herbs for emotional balance and harmony

Physical manifestations of illness are an expression of underlying dynamics, i.e. illness is always meaningful. Certain herbs can have a transformational action in a psycho-spiritual sense, that is they carry the influence of spirituality, which changes the nature of emotional experience. They have the capacity to transform a negative emotional impression into constructive spiritual virtue. This is a qualitative process which is not intellectually accessible.

Energetic actions of herbs

Certain herbs have a particular configuration which can 'inform' or bring into effect 'experience', 'patterning' or 'gestalts'. This is particularly applicable where there have been difficulties with role models or experiential gaps in development.

This approach is constructive, positive and contributory, and leads to self-empowerment. The energetic actions of herbs are related to their physical and physiological actions and are essentially a refinement or extension of feeling that emanates from the physical function. Restriction and congestion are associated with repressed emotion and impressions, which can be released, diffused or integrated with herbs. The resolution of emotional disturbance may require personal or spiritual growth, that is the person has to 'grow' bigger than the problem, this is the anticipated outcome of the therapeutic process involving the authentication of the patient through the patient–practitioner interaction and the intervention of the herbal medicine.

Flower essences and the development of the higher self

The life process is conceived as a process of the development of ones higher or spiritual self. Physical conditions states are seen as manifestations of the physical mind and as such are corporeal and separate us from who we really are. Flower essences are transformational remedies for self-mastery and development. Flower essences are based essentially on alchemy or transformational change where the symbolic representation of the goal of transformation is used as an agent for change.

Classification of herbal interventions

Nervous system restoratives	Avena sativa. Verbena officinalis. Hypericum perforatum. Scutellaria lateriflora. Turnera diffusa. Rosmarinus off. Stachys betonica. Tilia spp.
Nervous system balancers Stimulate, relax and restore. Provide a sense of connection or manifestation	Salvia officinalis. Rosmarinus officinalis. Hyssopus officinalis.
Integration and organisation	Centella asiatica. Tonics.
Interrelationships and interconnection (boundaries)	Achillea millefolium. Anemone pulsatilla. Angelica archangelica. Stachys betonica. Viola spp. Verbena officinalis.
Grounding and establishing foundation	Agrimonia eupatorium. Arctium lappa radix. Polygonum multiflorum. Tonics. Taraxacum officinale radix.
Relaxants	Chamomilla spp. Leonorus cardiac. Valeriana officinalis. Viburnum spp. Viscum alba.
Herbs for personal growth	Rosa spp. Citrus aurantium flores, Hyssopus officinale, Lavendula officinale. Ocimum spp. Viola spp. Verbena officinalis.

Herbs for nervous system

Herb	Therapeutic movement	Principal therapeutic actions
Avena sativa	Sweet. Warm. Moist. Nourishing and restoring.	Nervine tonic. Relaxant/antispasmodic. Sedative. Hyoglycaemic. Dermatological agent.
Citrus aurantium flores	Warm. Moist. Sweet. Bitter.	Antidepressant. Sedative. Antispasmodic. Carminative. Astringent. Bitter and cholagogue. Antiseptic.
Humulus lupulus	Cold. Dry. Bitter. Pungent. Astringent.	Sedative. CNS restorative. Antispasmodic. Analgesic. Hypnotic. Cholagogue. Hepatic. Anaphrodisiac. Oestrogenic. Antibacterial.
Hypericum perforatum	Cool. Dry. Bitter. Astringent. Relaxing, restorative.	Nerve Tonic. Antidepressant. Antibacterial. Antiviral. Anti-inflammatory. Vulnerary. Antihaemorrhagic.

Conditions applicable and combinations	Energetic actions and notes
Nervous debility and exhaustion. Sedative and relaxant for irritability, excitability, tremors, panic, insomnia. Affinity for the genitourinary system—PMS, bladder spasms, sexual hyperexcitability and impotence. Herpes zoster. Pruritic and inflamed dermatological conditions. **Special features: long term regenerative treatment for neurasthenia/debility.**	
Mood elevator. Insomnia. Sedative and spasmolytic for anxiety, tension and associated symptoms, e.g. nervous headache, dyspepsia. Hypertension and palpitations. Clears heat from the liver and associated organs. **Special features: a strong and uplifting tranquilliser.**	Clears emotional impressions and tension. A good facilitator.
Sedative and spasmolytic for GIT spasm, asthma, bladder spasm. Anxiety, irritability, tension, excitability. Sexual hyperexcitability. Dysmenorrhoea. Amenorrhoea. Menopause. Galactagogue. Insomnia. Digestive and liver stimulant—dyspepsia, nausea, constipation. Internalised heat conditions—eczema, furunculosis. Nematode infection. STDs **Special features: excitability associated with the GIT and reproductive system.** Insomnia with other remedies.	
Relaxing and tonic for anxiety, restlessness, depression, insomnia. Shock. Nerve injuries. Antispasmodic for GIT and genitourinary tract. Antiviral action against; Herpes 1 and 2, zoster. Epstein Barr etc. Reduces prolactin production. Hepatic protector. Topical—burns, blisters, wounds, tumours, herpes.	Essence is used as a protector for spiritual change.

(Continued)

Herb	Therapeutic movement	Principal therapeutic actions
Lavendula angustifolia	Cool. Dry. Bitter. Pungent. Dispersing, stimulating restoring.	Antidepressant. Relaxant. Sedative. Carminative. Stimulant. Cholagogue, choleretic. Antirheumatic.
Matricaria chamomilla/ Chamaemelum nobile	Cooling or warming. Calming. Bitter. Astringent.	Antispasmodic. Sedative. Anti-inflammatory. Antibacterial. Antifungal. Diaphorectic. Aromatic.
Passiflora incarnate	Cool. Dry.	Sedative. Antispasmodic. Hypnotic. Analgesic. Antibiotic. Antifungal. Hypotensive. Vasodilator.
Pelargonium graveolens	Cool. Moist. Clears heat and inflammation.	Antidepressant. Astringent. Anti-inflammatory. Haemostatic. Vulnerary. Aphrodisiac. Tonic.

Conditions applicable and combinations	Energetic actions and notes
Anxiety, depression. nervous irritability, insomnia. Spasm congestion associated with the GIT—colic, bloating, IBS. Nausea and vomiting. Motion sickness. Cerebral insufficiency—headache, migraine, memory, vertigo. Antineoplastic. Topical—anti-inflammatory, insect bites, dermatological agent, rubefacient, vulnerary, burns, neuralgia, strains and bruises. **Special features. balancing to the ANS—stimulates, relaxes and calms.**	Works on the higher CNS centres. For disharmony from shock and other invasion. General facilitator.
Anxiety, restlessness, insomnia. Antispasmodic for the GIT, respiratory and genitourinary systems. Headaches and migraines. Allergic reactions and membrane inflammation—respiratory, digestive, genital. Nausea and vomiting. Motion sickness. Amenorrhoea. Dysmenorrhoea. Eczema, dermatitis, impetigo, insect bites, burns, wounds. Teething pains, earache etc. in children. **Special features: antispasmodic and ani-inflammatory for all systems. Children's complaints.**	Matricaria may be more anti-inflammatory and Chamaemelum more sedating.
Anxiety. Agitation. Insomnia. Spasmolytic for GIT and respiratory systems. Excess sympathetic activity—hypertension, tachycardia. Drug addiction. **Special features: excess psychomotor activity. Insomnia.**	
Uplifting and relaxing for anxiety and depression, stress. Emotional tension associated with hormonal states—PMT, menopause. Aphrodisiac and adrenal tonic. Astringent for diarrhoea. Topical for sore throats as a gargle. Eczema **Special features: uplifting relaxant that has a restorative and nourishing action.**	

(Continued)

Herb	Therapeutic movement	Principal therapeutic actions
Piscidia erythrina	Cool. Dry. Bitter. Astringent.	Sedative. Hypnotic. Antispasmodic. Anti-inflammatory. Diaphoretic. Astringent. Diuretic. Antitussive.
Rosa damascena	Cold. Dry. Clears heat. Restores and nourishes.	Antidepressant. Sedative. Astringent. Anti-inflammatory. Hepatic, cholagogue. Anticholesterolaemic. Aphrodisiac. Antipyretic. Antiviral.
Scutellaria laterifolia	Cold. Dry. Bitter. Astringent.	Antispasmodic. Sedative. Nerve. Tonic. Anti-inflammatory. Anodyne. Anticonvulsant.
Stachys betonica	Cold. Dry. Bitter. Astringent. Scatters wind heat.	Tonic. Antispasmodic. Cerebral. Stimulant. Alterative. Astringent. Hepatic.

Conditions applicable and combinations	Energetic actions and notes
Sedative and spasmolytic for anxiety, tension. Insomnia. Neuralgia. Antitussive and antispasmodic for asthma, pertussis etc. Sciatica. Neuralgia. Diarrhoea. Intestinal spasm. **Special features: insomnia and associated neurasthenia.**	
Relaxing and uplifting for anxiety and depression. Cleansing, tonic and restorative to the liver. Clears liver and blood heat—eczema, dermatitis. Menorrhagia, metrorrhagia, uterine fibroids. Hormonally associated emotional upset depression. Aphrodisiac. Fertility enhancer. Antiviral agent, HIV. Laxative, especially for children. Astringent and anti-inflammatory for mouth ulcers, gingivitis, conjunctivitis. Topical—radiation burns, dermatitis.	For 'coming to terms' emotionally.
Nervous restlessness, excitability, panic, anxiety, insomnia, obsession. Nerve restorative for weak, debilitated, sensitive systems. Deliriuim tremens. Hysteria. Epilepsy. Convulsions. Muscular spasms and tremors. Hypertension. Clears heat and toxins from the liver and kidneys **Special features: a relaxing and sedating herb with long term benefits of tonification and strengthening.**	Particularly effective for working with anxiety associated with deep patterns of trauma.
Cerebral tonic and restorative—memory, concentration, headache, vertigo. Eye problems from deficiency—cataract, conjunctivitis, poor eye sight.	Enables a connection and expression to be made between emotional repressions and conscious experience.

(Continued)

Herb	Therapeutic movement	Principal therapeutic actions
Valeriana officinalis	Warm. Dry. Bitter. Pungent.	Antispasmodic. Sedative. Hypnotic. Hypotensive. Antibacterial.
Verbena officinalis	Cool. Dry. Bitter. Astringent. Eliminative. Restorative. Diffusive.	ANS Relaxant. Tonic. Bitter. Cholagogue. Diaphoretic. Antidepressant. Emmenagogue. Galactagogue.
Viscum album	Cold. Moist.	Antispasmodic, sedative, tonic. Hypotensive. Haemostatic.

Conditions applicable and combinations	Energetic actions and notes
Anxiety. Panic attacks. GIT relaxant and tonic. Cleansing action on the liver—rheumatism, sciatica. Astringent, healing action on mucous membranes. Diarrhoea. Haemostatic. Vulnerary. **Special features: a relaxing and stimulating herb that removes toxaemia and stasis from the viscera and encourages the upward and outward flow of blood and energy. Has long term regenerative action.**	
Anxiety, tension, excitability. Headache. Migraine. Insomnia. Antispasmodic for GIT. **Special features: to relax smooth muscle constriction attendant upon anxiety. Mental clarity is unaffected at moderate doses.**	Do not use where there is mania.
Spasmodic nervine and antidepressant for debilitated nervous conditions. Anxiety, insomnia, irritability. Stimulant and tonic to the liver, gall bladder and GIT, removing heat and toxicity. Antispasmodic for asthma, bronchitis, sinus problems. Amenorrhoea, dysmenorrhoea—tones and cleanses the uterus. Urinary tract spasm, dysuria, gravel. Aphrodisiac. **Special features: relaxing, cleansing, astringing tonic for the viscera—removing obstructions and facilitating a diffusive and externalising action.**	For the tension and scattered disharmony associated with over striving, anxiety and competitiveness.
Relaxant for anxiety, tension, panic attacks. Antispasmodic for hypertension. Cardiac tonic. Immune stimulant. Anticancer. Uterine stimulant and antihemorrhagic (post-partum). **Special features: excess parasympathetic nerve activity. Antidepressant withdrawal.**	

Case history: anxiety

This patient is a 26-year-old administrator. She feels as though she has the symptoms of anxiety. She feels stressed and during the day feels very tense, especially in her lungs. She often has a muzzy head and sense of dislocation. She has significant fatigue, especially in the mornings and at weekends and usually spends them in her pyjamas. Her peripheral circulation is cold and sometimes she is cold to the core but has no night heat.

Menstrual cycle (MC): slightly short recently, some spotting with ovulation and some dysmenorrhoea. No PMS.

This woman is fashionably dressed and well-groomed. She is sociable, articulate and with good interpersonal skills. She is a graduate, temporarily working as an administrator whilst considering her future career. She is married but recently separated from her husband.

Clinical signs:
Blood pressure: 126/90.
Pulse: 60.
Pulse pressure: 36.
Tongue: pale and swollen, slightly slippery, cracking in the tip.

Herb	Dosage	Physiological actions	Energetic actions
Angelica sinensis	15.00	Blood and hormone tonic. Spasmolytic.	Protective. Sense of calm and peace.
Centella	15.00	ANS/CNS balancer. Tonic. Restorative.	Authority and control.
Codonopsis	20.00	Foundational tonic.	Sense of authority. Foundation.
Astragalus	15.00	Promotion of immunological protection. Tonic.	
Schizandra	10.00	Tonic facilitator.	Free movement of the fire principal.
Iris	10.00	Liver tonic and adaptogen.	Expression of creativity and inspiration.
Rosa	10.00	Liver tonic. Emotional tone.	Self-embrace and esteem.
Glycyrrhiza	15.00	Nourishing foundational tonic.	Nourishment of self.
Borago	20.00	Adrenal tonification.	Courage and resolve.
Stachys	15.00	Cerebral-spinal regulator. Nerve tonic.	Autonomic balance and regulation.
Rosmarinus officinalis	10.00	ANS balancer. Restorative. Aromatic.	Manifestation of self.
Dosage: 5 ml bid.	155.00		

Differential diagnosis:
Anaemia. Hypothyroidism. Chronic fatigue syndrome. The patient has a significant deficiency in cardiovascular output—with a pulse pressure of 36 and a pulse rate of 60, despite the consultation taking place in the middle of the day whilst at work, when you normally expect sympathetic activation. A pulse of 60, without indications of significant involvement in exercise, is indicative of a slow metabolic rate, which could be indicative of hypothyroidism or subclinical hypothyroidism, associated with a significant fatigue syndrome. It is noted that she can be 'cold to the core' and easily gains weight, both significant to a low metabolic rate. Notably, when not at work, her energy levels are very low.

The patient was questioned about the difference between the experience of anxiety and the experience of the symptoms of anxiety. She felt that psychologically she wasn't anxious but felt the consequences of anxiety in her body. This could be an important distinction as a significant deficiency condition gives rise to a feeling of vulnerability and anxiety which may not be felt to be coherent to her circumstances.

She is demonstrating significant sympathetic deficiency and smooth muscle constraint, which could be indicative that she is in a situation that she finds difficult and perhaps where she has problematical boundaries. It is possible that she has not had a strong authentication experience from a male role model and hence has an element of disconnection or unreality.

Her autonomic dysfunction could relate to her recent break up with her husband and that she is temporally staying with her brother. She revealed that she found her current work tedious within a firm where there are significant stresses and tensions. Questioning revealed that she has an artistic inclination and feels unfulfilled. She is thinking of going travelling and teaching English as a foreign language.

The herbal intervention is designed to provide:

- A deep nourishing action to improve her foundation, hormonal status and blood and consequently her sense of stability and integrity
- Enable resilience, flexibility and determination in her boundaries
- Provide clarity of purpose in her decision making
- Engender authentication and value of her personal self

Case history: anxiety

This 37-year-old housewife suffers from generalised anxiety and intermittent panic attacks, which she has had for some two years. The symptoms were apparently triggered by routine surgery. She reported relatively normal well-being previously. She has no particular concerns with her marriage or family life. She reports her energy to be poor. She feels vulnerable, fragmented and disorientated.

Clinical signs:
Blood pressure: 90/60.
Pulse: 104.
Pulse pressure: 30.

CVI: 15,600.
Tongue: Pale, swollen body with heat in the tip.
Blood tests reveal no abnormalities.

Analysis and interpretation:
The clinical signs show a significant deficiency, as demonstrated by the low pulse pressure. The pulse is high, which is probably compensatory (blood tests mitigate against pathophysiological causes). It is difficult to determine to what extent this is primarily psychosomatic shock due to an existential crisis created by the trauma and invasion of surgery or whether the trauma precipitated the manifestation of an underlying fatigue syndrome. The patient stated that she wanted an urgent and effective intervention and was not likely to be compliant with a long-term and progressive treatment.

Herb	Physiological actions	Energetic actions
Stachys betonica	Cerebral-spinal regulator. Nerve tonic.	Autonomic balance and regulation.
Verbena officinalis	Nerve tonic and restorative.	Self-affirmation and strength.
Rosmarinus officinalis	ANS balancer. Restorative. Aromatic	Restore cerebral blood circulation.
Rosa damascena	Liver tonic. Emotional tone.	Self-esteem and safety.
Valeriana officinalis	Nerve relaxant.	Sense of tranquillity.
Flower essences: Agrimony, Cherry Plum, Walnut, Holly, Crab Apple		Acceptance. Letting go. Protection from outside influences. Freedom from hurt. Purity.

Rationale:
The aim of the medicine was to quickly improve the cerebral circulation with cerebral restoratives and to underpin the action with autonomic regulation, stability and reassurance. The medicine worked within one day. She took the medicine for a month and then discontinued without the reoccurrence of symptoms.

Case history: obsessive-compulsive disorder

A 42-year-old former bank clerk and now housewife and mother of two children, aged 8 and 6, has been in her current relationship for 11 years and married for two months. This lady has an obsessive cleaning disorder, which has been worsening for the past few years. She has always been very concerned with cleaning and always kept a very clean house, but she is aware that the situation is becoming disruptive and she particularly does not want to create problems for her children as they become older. She frequently washes her hands between simple tasks, requests that her children and her husband wash their hands as soon as they come in, washes the children's clothes every day or twice a day if they have been out, washes the toilet twice a day etc. She is worried that herself, her children and her house may become contaminated.

Previous medical history:
She has a history of viral infections; herpes, German measles, shingles and, at the age of 15, glandular fever. From June 1994 she developed ME and became increasingly physically and mentally exhausted with muscular weakness and pain, poor concentration, tinnitus and anxiety and depression. She recovered following treatment with herbal medicine and Bach flower essences. The turning point came when she experienced a traumatic re-experience of a family house fire, which occurred when she was 12. This occurred during the night and she re-experienced the terror she had felt at the time, together with the experience of the smoke, panic etc. The following day on waking she was free from her symptoms of ME.

She has had a tendency to suffer from agoraphobia to a greater or lesser extent all of her life. When she worked in a bank she was an extremely hard worker and worked far harder than strictly necessary and was extremely conscientious.

Physical symptoms:
She reports feeling tense and anxious. She says her energy is good. She feels the cold.

Orthodox medicine:
Thyroxine, 100 μmg for ten years. Contraceptive pill.

Clinical signs:
Blood pressure: 120/85.
Pulse: 80.
Pulse pressure: 35.
Tongue: pale and swollen with disparate papillae in the anterior one-third and a slippery coating.

She appears tense, with a shiny pale complexion and fishy eyes.

Family history:
She is the middle of three daughters and was told that she was the favourite child. She felt that she was always striving to be good, so that she would deserve her mother's affection, and used to spend much time cleaning her room and moving the furnishings around. Her mother was and continues to be very critical. She feels as if she has never had her own life, but it has been shared with her mother. This control has continued since moving to her own house and since her marriage. Critical comments are never made if the husband is present and she will check when she is telephoning whether he is within ear shot. If she complains her mother tells her not to be so sensitive, she is only telling her what she needs to know.

When she was very young she remembers her parents having frequent arguments and although she didn't witness any violence she remembers being worried that her father would hit her mother. This also became a recurring dream over a period of years. She remembers her mother shaking and trembling and pouring herself a drink to steady herself.

Analysis:
There is an ANS imbalance, which expresses lack of control and authority. Parental behaviour should demonstrate consistent love and concern, together with acceptance and recognition of the growing independence and autonomy and affirm the essential integrity of the child. This creates a context of self-acceptance and authority, which becomes internalised and accepted as a reality by the unconscious processes of the child. The fundamental belief in one's own integrity and worth means that the person, as an adult, will always act in their own best interests and broadcast this message to those in their immediate environment, maintain appropriate boundaries, and feel safe and relaxed. She has not been able to, or shown how, to break the ties with her mother and establish a proper relationship, and her mother continues to control and manipulate her daughter and rely on her as a support system.

Herb	*Physiological actions*	*Energetic actions*
Achillea millefolium	Circulatory facilitator.	Promotion of effective boundaries.
Panax ginseng	Foundational tonic.	Sense of authority and strength in one's self.
Schizandra	Adjunct for tonics.	Circulation of the 'fire' principle.
Hydrastis canadensis	Tissue restorative. Liver heat.	Transformative agent for personal change.
Paeonia	Liver tonic and restorative.	Engenders deep sense of femininity.
Polygonum multiflorum	Foundation tonic for the vital organs and nervous system.	
Hypericum perfoliatum	Trophorestorative for the nervous system.	Facilitator for personal transformation.
Rosamarinus officinalis	ANS tonic and regulator.	Affirmation and manifestation of self.
Citrus aurantium flores	CNS tranquiliser.	Maintenance of calm in difficult circumstances.
Flower essences: Cherry Plum, Crab Apple Centaury, Rock Rose, Walnut, Holly, Star of Bethylhem	Letting go. Personal distaste. Shock. Self-assertion and promotion. Protection against external interference.	

The cardiovascular system

The heart

Cardiovascular disease

The relationship between cholesterol and arterial disease is unclear, although mainstream medicine regards cholesterol as a key factor. Although the evidence is that statins reduce cholesterol levels, it has not been demonstrated that the reduction of cholesterol reduces the incidence of cardiovascular disease. In fact, there is some evidence that moderate levels of cholesterol are protective. Hyperglyceridaemia associated with high blood glucose levels may be more important and is not necessarily related to hypercholesterolemia. It is certainly the case that hyperglycaemia is a major contributory cause and the key factors for hyperglycaemia are calorie overload, lack of exercise, stress and inflammation, and endocrine disorders. Exercise and reduced calories improve high density lipoproteins/low density lipoproteins ratios and hyperglycaemia. The factors of the states of deficiency, depletion and congestion are always important and need to be identified and addressed. Congestion of the liver is implicated, in particular and associated with conditions of toxicity and poor tissue healing and integrity.

Hypertension

In mainstream medicine, hypertension is seen as intrinsically linked with cardiovascular disease, to the extent that hypertension is regarded as a causative factor. This view is, however, changing and risk factors for cardiovascular disease are considered as hyperglycaemia, high BMI, lack of exercise, smoking and hypertension. It would certainly be the case that in cardiovascular disease, there is likely to be an increase in blood pressure, necessary to overcome the resistance of vascular tissue degeneration. Although, in advanced cardiovascular degeneration, the blood pressure falls due to a lack of arterial tissue tone. Hypertension may also be related in some circumstances to inflammatory and stress factors, both of which are implicated in the generation of cardiovascular disease.

The diagnosis of essential hypertension suggests that there is no known cause. From the perspective of herbal therapeutics, a number of factors may apply (see section on The interpretation of clinical signs):

- Hormone deficiency may cause vascular tension through the induction of smooth muscle constriction. Rises in blood pressure often follow hormone deficiency states, e.g. menopause.
- Smooth muscle constriction may relate to reflex 'guarding' or emotional tension. This is an autonomic flinch mechanism.
- The systolic and diastolic is affected by stress, a mechanism similar to the flinch mechanism mentioned above, together with sympathetic activation and is a consequence of autonomic vigilance to anticipated danger.
- The relationship between the systolic and diastolic, i.e. the pulse pressure demonstrates the balance of the ANS. The sympathetic tone, and hence the blood pressure, frequently rises as a compensatory mechanism for fatigue factors and symptomatic reduction doesn't serve a particularly useful purpose.
- Cardiovascular health is a major factor. Blood pressure may increase as a compensatory mechanism for poor vascular tissue state. With advanced cardiovascular disease, the blood pressure often falls due to decreased elasticity and tone of the vascular tissue.
- High sodium may be implicated but is controversial. Insulin resistance causes sodium retention and, hence, increased blood volume. Low potassium and magnesium, and possibly low calcium, affect blood pressure.

Symptomatic treatment of blood pressure is inherently problematical, as it doesn't address the aetiological causes and therefore may cause significant side effects. In clinical practice, it is not unusual to find a situation where blood pressure may be increased by medication, i.e. where the physiological response to treatment is to endeavour to overcome the effects of a reduction in pressure, further medication compounds the problem. Treatment protocols should address core problems and will most likely address a number of factors at the same time, e.g. hormone deficiency, foundation energy depletion, compromised tissue states and inflammation and stress factors. It is to be noted that changes in blood pressure are usual when treating constitutionally, i.e. when core issues are being addressed.

Metabolic syndrome

Metabolic syndrome is a common and potentially serious condition, which can be seen as a precursor to cardiovascular disease. In addition to dietary indiscretions it is linked to stress factors and adrenal fatigue.

Diagnostic criteria:

- HDL cholesterol of less than 40 mg/dL in men or less than 50 mg/dL in women
- Triglyceride level of 150 mg/dL or greater

- Abdominal obesity
- Systolic blood pressure (top number) of 130 mm Hg or greater
- Diastolic blood pressure of 85 mm Hg or greater
- Fasting glucose of 100 mg/dL or greater
- Metabolic syndrome is closely associated with insulin resistance. For people who suffer from this condition, their bodies can't use insulin efficiently. Therefore, metabolic syndrome is also called insulin resistance syndrome.
- Magnesium. Insulin stores magnesium and with insulin resistance magnesium cannot be stored and is excreted. Magnesium relaxes smooth muscle.
- Fructose is metabolised into a number of waste products, including uric acid. Uric acid inhibits nitric oxide, which relaxes smooth muscle and helps blood vessels maintain their elasticity (Longmore et al., 2014).

The peripheral circulation

- Tissue perfusion is less reliant on arterial integrity and efficiency than on factors that affect tissue diffusion—the condition of the capillary wall, the action of vasoactive agents, such as pro-inflammatory factors and histamine, and congestion within the lymphatic and venous systems.
- Raynaud's disease—consequent of spasm in the terminal arterioles mediated be a spinal reflex. Raynaud's is closely associated with inflammation. Poor peripheral circulation may be a less acute manifestation, or may relate to the balance of the ANS and system circulation, and is closely related to endogenous heat.
- Cerebral circulatory deficiency symptomatically presents as unsteadiness, dizziness, dull headache, fogginess, problems with memory and concentration.
- Related to poor peripheral circulation.
- May have a number of causes:
  - Sympathetic nerve deficiency with accompanying high diastolic tone, i.e. low pulse pressure
  - Congestion of the blood in the internal organs, in particular liver congestion
  - Arteriosclerotic changes
  - Qualitative problems with the blood, e.g. anaemia
  - Quantitative issues of the blood, e.g. blood volume
- Cerebral circulatory deficiency may relate to a feeling of tension and restriction in the neck, shoulders and back of head, affecting the basilar artery—may present as TIA or arthritis.
- Ulceration is a common manifestation of poor arterial circulation and venous stasis.

Herbs for cardiovascular health

Herbs for the treatment of arterial disease have complex actions which include regulation of fat and sugar metabolism, cleansing, restoring and nourishing the endothelium, antioxidant and anti-inflammatory properties.

Condition	Therapeutic intervention
Heart disease. Herbs to regulate and improve myocardial efficiency.	Convallaria majalis. Selenicerus grandifolia. Crataegus spp.
Arterial relaxants and peripheral dilators. Antispasmodics.	Crataegus spp. Viburnum opulus, Leonorus cardiac. Achillea millefolium. Tilia spp. Viscum alba. Gingko biloba. Angelica archangelica. Crataegus, Viburnum opulus, Viscum alba. Zanthoxylum americanum. Zingiberis officinalis.
Palpitations. Functional tachycardia or palpitations should be differentiated from arrhythmia arising from problems of heart conduction—heart block, atrial fibrillation. The vagal nerve largely controls heart rate. Causative factors: • Anxiety or emotional stress through action on the ANS—sympathetic deficiency. • Reflex disturbance from the digestive function—wind and bloating. • Action of hormone deficiency or imbalance on the ANS, e.g. hyperthyroidism, menopause, PMS. • Deficiency of magnesium, calcium. • Dietary excess of foods containing adrenal-activating substances (coffee, cheese, chocolate etc.). • Drugs and herbs with sympathomimetic action.	Tonics to lift the sympathetic tone of the autonomic nervous system. Seleniferous grandifolia is specific for functional palpitation from sympathetic deficiency. Leonorus cardiac. Anemone pulsatilla. Lycopus virginicus. Crataegus spp. Chamomilla recutita, Melissa officinalis. Lavendula officinalis.

Actions	Herbal intervention
Arterial restoratives.	Depuratives and hepatics. Anti-inflammatories. Allium spp. Curcuma longa. Cynara scolymus. Tilia spp. Taraxacum officinalis radix. Althaea officinale.
Cerebral-spinal restoratives: To improve and restore cerebral circulation and the balance of the autonomic response.	Tonics, circulatory herbs. Rosmarinus, Stachys, Carbenia, Schizandra, Gingko.
Endothelial tissue healing.	Calendula officinalis. Achillea millefolium. Centella asiatica. Equisetum arvensis.

The venous system

Problems in the venous system may be evidenced by back pressure causing haemorrhoids and varicose veins. Varices associated with other organs may occur but not be evidenced, e.g. oesophageal varices associated with liver disease. This may not be recognised until advanced, oesophageal varices from liver disease are an important cause of haemoptysis.

Causes of haemorrhoids and varicose veins include pelvic obstruction, e.g. pregnancy, pelvic congestion through circulatory dysfunction and visceroptosis, congestion of the portal circulation consequent upon stagnation of liver function, deficiency of tissue integrity of the vein walls.

Actions	Herbal intervention
Tonics to improve vascular tone.	Aesculus hippocastanum. Ruscus aculeatus. Crataegus spp.
Circulatory herbs for venous circulation.	Achillea millefoliu. Myrica.
Hepatic portal circulation.	Hepatics. Specific: Collinsonia canadensis. Taraxacum officinale radix.
Astringent and anti-inflammatory herbs for local application.	Symphytum officinale. Calendula officinalis. Hamamaelis virginicana.
Internal and external applications for haemorrhoids.	Ranunculus ficaria. Hamamaelis virginicana.

Factors for improving cardiovascular health

Carbohydrate load and sugar optimisation	Reduce calorie intake especially refined carbohydrates. A cyclical ketogenic diet as far as possible.
Whole food diet	Nutrient dense foods including, eggs, butter and other healthy fats. Fruit, vegetables, nuts and seeds.
Optimise fat intake	Omega 3, especially from low mercury oily fish. Minimise industrially produced oils and foods.
Healthy sun exposure	Optimises vitamin D. Nitric oxide production. Ensure against burning.
Exercise	Regulate cardiovascular, non-exhaustive, exercise.
Inflammatory drivers	Treat infections. Treat inflammatory factors and endogenous heat.
Healthy blood pressure	Stress reduction. A mindset of optimism and acceptance.

- Many of the herbs in this category are classified as diaphoretics, i.e. are used to induce sweating in the treatment of fevers, to equalise the circulation and to promote cleansing through the skin.
- Circulate blood and energy in an upward and outward movement.
- Energetically are associated with protective and cleansing qualities.

Herbs for the circulatory system

Herb	Therapeutic movement	Principal therapeutic actions
Convallaria majalis	Stimulating, restoring, dissolving. Bitter. Sweet.	Cardiac tonic and restorative. Spasmolytic. Anti-inflammatory. Nerve restorative.
Crataegus spp.	Resolving, decongesting, restoring. Bitter. Astringent. Sweet.	Cardiac and circulatory tonic and restorative. Antioxidant. Spasmolytic and sedative. Decongestant. Parasympathetic restorative and balancer.
Leonorus cardiaca	Relaxing, restoring. Bitter. Pungent. Cool.	Stimulating and relaxing antispasmodic.
Selenicerous grandifloria	Stimulating, restoring, resolving. Bitter. Sweet. Cool.	Stimulating, regulating, balancing and restorative tonic for cardiac function and ANS. Thyroactive. Restores sympathetic tone.
Tilia spp.	Relaxing, dissolving. Pungent. Sweet. Astringent.	Relaxing, sedating and antispasmodic action. Diaphoretic.
Viscum album	Cold.	Stimulating, relaxing and antispasmodic for the ANS and cardiac function. Restores parasympathetic function Immunological stimulant.

Circulatory herbs

Herb	Therapeutic movement	Principal therapeutic actions
Achillea millefolium	Diaphoretic. Astringent. Bitter. Sweet. Dry. Decongesting, resolving.	Astringent. Anti-inflammatory. Depurative. Haemostatic. Bitter. Antibiotic. Antispasmodic, carminative. Cholagogue, choleretic.

Conditions applicable and combinations	Energetic actions and notes
Cardiac deficiency, angina, cardiac failure. Oedema from cardiac and circulatory deficiency. Hypotension. Palpitations. Congestive heart failure.	Small quantities with Leonorus and Crataegus.
Degenerative and deficient conditions of cardiac function—angina, myocardial insufficiency. Coronary heart disease. Arterial disease. Palpitations. Anxiety and anguish particularly associated with hormone deficiency.	Central energy decongestant with associated calming and reassuring action.
Relaxing, balancing, regulating and restorative action on the uterus and heart. Dysmenorrhoea, amenorrhoea, pre-menstrual tension. Cardiac deficiency, palpitations. Hyperthyroid and hypertension.	Balances the heart-uterus dynamic.
Cardiac deficiency and debility states. Antidepressant and nerve restorative. Contraindicated in excess conditions, e.g. hypertension.	Apprehension or foreboding associated with danger or death.
Depression, agitation, nervous tension, restlessness. Hypertension, dyspnoea, headache. Arteriosclerosis. Sympathetic resolvent.	
Excess cardiac conditions—hypertension, angina, congestive headache. Symptoms arising from hormone deficiency—post menopausal syndromes aggravated by tension. Hysteria, epilepsy. Cancer. Chronic arthritis. Neuritis.	

Conditions applicable and combinations	Energetic actions and notes
A stimulating and relaxing remedy, improves the circulation of blood and energy and improves the condition of the tissues of the circulation. A tonic restorative for the mucous membranes.	Pregnancy.

(Continued)

Herb	Therapeutic movement	Principal therapeutic actions
Anemone pulsatilla	Warm. Dry. Slightly bitter and pungent. Relaxing and stimulating.	Antispasmodic nervine. Stimulant. Diaphoretic. Antiseptic, antibacterial. Anti-inflammatory. Diuretic. Emmenagogue.
Angelica archangelica Herba/radix Also: Angelica sinensis Andgelica dehurica	Warm. Dry. Bitter. Pungent. Sweet. Restoring, stimulating and relaxing.	A stimulating and relaxing diffusive tonic. Antispasmodic, carminative. Antibacterial, antifungal, antiseptic. Bitter. Diuretic. Cholagogue.
Crataegus oxyacanthoides Berry Flower tops	Decongesting. Cool. Dry. Astringent. Bitter. Sweet.	Cardiac restorative and tonic. Spasmolytic and sedative. Astringent.
Eupatorium perfoliatum	Dry. Cool. Astringent. Bitter. Pungent.	Diaphoretic. Anti-inflammatory. Antispasmodic. Expectorant.
Ginkgo biloba		Circulatory stimulant. Anti-inflammatory. Antioxidant. Immunostimulant.
Nepeta cataria	Cool. Dry. Bitter. Pungent. Aromatic.	Diaphoretic. Antispasmodic. Aromatic. Carminative. Analgesic.

Conditions applicable and combinations	Energetic actions and notes
Anxiety, irritability, tension, panic attacks, hysterical reactions, insomnia as a relaxant and sedative. Nervous exhaustion. Cold, deficient circulation. Tachycardia. Hypertension. Antispasmodic for asthma, bronchitis, pertussis. Affinity for the special sense organs; antispasmodic, anodyne, anti-catarrhal. Painful conditions of the male and female reproductive systems; ovaritis, dysmenorrhoea, amenorrhoea, prostatitis, prostatic hypertrophy, orchitis. Impotence and sexual dysfunction from over excitability and anxiety. Chickenpox, measles to clear toxins and support the CNS. Furunculosis.	A strong spasmolytic with many applications. In an energetic sense may be related to its common name the wind flower, i.e. is stabilising in agitated, confused and disturbed conditions.
Circulatory insufficiency. Vascular disease—Intermittent claudication. Headache and migraine. Respiratory infections, bronchitis, coughs, asthma. Dyspepsia. Appetite stimulant. Alcoholism. Menopausal symptoms.	Protective and opening. Emphasis on the head and higher centres. Caution: Pregnancy. Photosensitisation. Inflammation of the GIT.
Circulatory insufficiency. Regulating, restoring and tonic to the heart. Regulates function and improves efficiency of myocardium.	Vascular decongestant. Opens and soothes the emotional 'heart'.
Chronic catarrh, bronchitis, pneumonia. Bitter relaxant for the liver. Laxative. **Special features: stimulating and relaxing diaphoretic for the outward circulation of blood and energy in chronic conditions. For pyrexia in acute respiratory infection—colds, flu.**	
Circulatory insufficiency especially cerebral. Headaches, tinnitus. vertigo, Alzheimer's macular degeneration and glaucoma vascular disease—intermittent claudication, temporal arteritis, thrombosis, CVA. Asthma. **Special features: vasotonic and protective action to the vascular system. Has an amphoteric action to regulate circulatory function.**	
Dyspepsia, colic, flatus, spasm. Insomnia. Panic attacks, anxiety, hysteria. Amenorrhoea, Dysmenorrhoea, PMT.	

(Continued)

Herb	Therapeutic movement	Principal therapeutic actions
Sambucus nigra	Dry. Bitter. Sweet. Pungent.	Diaphoretic. Anti-inflammatory. Depurative. Antiallergic. Diuretic. Laxative.
Tilia spp.	Cool. Dry. Astringent. Sweet. Pungent.	Circulatory stimulant. Diaphoretic. Antispasmodic and sedative. Astringent. Demulcent.

Case history: hypertension

This lady, aged 69, presents with hypertension. Her GP had become concerned about her blood pressure and has doubled her medication. Her blood pressure was measured in the surgery at 180/96 with a pulse of 84. Generally, she is symptom free but gets a headache in the afternoons. She describes her energy as variable but low in the mornings and improves with exercise. She used to be cold but now describes herself as warm.

She describes herself as sensitive and has a reaction to many foods and medicines. She is intolerant to grains and dairy foods. She describes herself as easily psychologically overwhelmed and compromised. The patient had breast cancer four years ago, which was treated by a lumpectomy. She has had a reoccurrence near to the same site for approximately one year, for which she is not taking any treatment.

Orthodox medicine: Bisoprolol. Felodipine.

Clinical signs:
Blood pressure: 180/90
Pulse: 66.
Pulse pressure: 90.
Tongue: red, swollen base, crack towards the tip of the tongue.

The clinical signs show diastolic tension. This may be due to hormone deficiency, in part, but would be significant to a constraint pattern typical of a sensitive personality. The patient is

Conditions applicable and combinations	Energetic actions and notes
Pyrexia. **Special features: relaxing and soothing diaphoretic for the over excited nervous system. Nervous headache.**	
Chronic respiratory catarrh, rhinitis, sinusitis, laryngitis. Dyspepsia, colic, flatus. To cool hot blood conditions—eczema, dermatitis, psoriasis, measles etc. **Special features: relaxing and cleansing tonic depurative for circulatory insufficiency and congestion.**	
Migraine, headache. Upper respiratory catarrh and infection. **Special features: a relaxing and restoring diaphoretic for vascular disease to improve vascular flow and restore tissue integrity, e.g. arteriosclerosis. Hypertension. As a gentle relaxant and sedative for insomnia, hyperactivity and restlessness.**	Specific for excessive sympathetic tone, particularly in the vascular system.

clearly very concerned about her blood pressure, and also about what she considers to be a heroic treatment, and the stress is probably contributing to her blood pressure. It is possible that the elevated systolic pressure may be a response to the medication, an attempt by the body to compensate for the actions of the medicines.

Therapeutic aims:
Embodiment. Personal control and regulation.

Herb	Physiological actions	Energetic actions
Crataegus	Cardiovascular health	
Centella	Adaptogen. CNS and ANS regulator. Anti-inflammatory. Anxiolytic and antidepressant (Gohil et al. 2010).	Control and regulation.
Eucommia	Foundation tonic. Connective tissue tonic. Hypertension from sympathetic compensation for fatigue.	Strength of foundation.

(Continued)

Herb	Physiological actions	Energetic actions
Schizandra	Adjunct for tonics and adaptogens.	Movement of 'fire'.
Cimicifuga	Cerebral-spinal restorative. Nerve tonic.	
Stachys	Nerve tonic.	Autonomic regulation of the psycho-social interconnection.
Verbena	Nerve tonic and restorative.	Self-affirmation and strength.
Rosa	Liver heat. Nervine.	Emotional resolution.
Flower essences: Agrimony. Cherry Plum. Walnut. Rock Rose. Holly.	Acceptance. Trust. Protection. Resolve.	
Iris (addition)	Hepatic.	Promotion of female creativity and receptivity.

Two weeks:
Blood pressure: 172/88.
Home blood pressure: 149/78.

Six weeks:
Blood pressure: 152/90.
Pulse: 62.
Calmer. More energy and coping better.

Case history: cardiovascular disease

This 70 year old man suffered a myocardial infarction five years previously and he now has atrial fibrillation and angina attacks once or twice a week. He has low energy. His digestion is poor, with rabbit dropping stools, wind and bloating, acid indigestion and a queasy sensation. He feels dull-headed with a tight band around his temples and he has a stiff neck and shoulders. His peripheral circulation is cold.

Clinical signs:
Blood pressure: 155/100.
Pulse: 76.
Pulse pressure: 55.
CVI: 19,380.
Tongue: swollen, central flexure, white greasy coating, anterior heat papillae.

Analysis and interpretation:
It is a concern that despite an elevated CVI, this man is still significantly deficient, i.e. he has overactivity of his digestive function and poor cerebral circulation, suggesting low sympathetic activation but excess parasympathetic activation. There is probably a combination of significant psychogenic constraints causing smooth muscle constriction and significant cardiovascular disease creating circulatory impediment. A CVI of 19,380 suggests an adrenergic stress response, probably as a compensatory activating response. The emphasis for the therapeutic intervention is on the prevention of further cardiovascular incidence. Agents are used to improve myocardial function, i.e. Achillea, Crataegus, Leonorus and Convallaria; to improve arterial microcirculation and tissue integrity, i.e. Symphytum, Equisetum and Tilia; and to improve his energy foundation, i.e. Polygonum and Symphytum.

Herb	Dosage	Actions
Achillea millefolium	15.00	Diffusive peripheral circulatory vasodilator. Anti-inflammatory. Tissue restorative. Antispasmodic.
Crataegus oxy. berry	15.00	Heart and cardiovascular restorative. Coronary vasodilator. Antispasmodic. Hypotensive. Adaptogenic, restorative and decongestant.
Convallaria majalis	10.00	Regulates and strengthens cardiac function.
Leonorus cardiaca	15.00	Relaxant and antispasmodic for the heart and nerves. Hypotensive.
Polygonum multiflorum radix	30.00	Foundational and restorative tonic.
Symphytum officinale herba	15.00	Tissue healer and restorative. Foundational nutritional tonic.
Equisetum arvensis	15.00	Anti-atheroma. Tissue astringent, restorative and remineraliser.
Tilia spp.	30.00	Anti-atheroma. Anti-coagulant. Diaphoretic. Hypotensive.
Zanthoxylum clavaherculis fructus	5.00	Diffusive stimulant to the arterial, peripheral and cerebral circulation. Antispasmodic.
Dosage: 5 ml bid aq ac.	150.00	

Case history: cerebral circulatory deficiency

This lady of 72, complains of a dull, low grade headache, which starts upon rising in the morning and continues for most of the day. She is very fatigued, stressed and feels fragile. She has arthritis in her hips, knees and wrists. Her husband, who was 20 years her senior, died 18 months previously. She had been his carer for a number of years due to his poor health.

Clinical signs:
Blood pressure: 100/60.
Pulse: 74.
Pulse pressure: 40.
CVI: 11,840.
Tongue: pale and swollen with slight cracking to the surface.

Analysis:
The relatively low pulse pressure and CVI are indicative of passive sympathetic deficiency, which would be expected after the death of the person for whom one has long been the carer, and is the consequence of a post-traumatic fatigue syndrome and emotional distress. Morning fatigue and deficient cerebral circulation are typical of endocrine depletion. The formulation is to provide foundational support and recovery of the sympathetic tone and normal autonomic functioning.

Herb	Dosage	Actions
Angelica sinensis	20.00	Blood and hormone tonic. Relaxant and restorative.
Panax ginseng	15.00	Foundational tonic and adaptogen.
Schizandra chinensis	10.00	Tonic adjunct and facilitator.
Polygonum multiflorum radix	20.00	Foundational and restorative tonic.
Rehmannia glutinosa prep	20.00	Nutritional foundational tonic for the endocrines system, especially the adrenal cortex.
Rosamarinus officinale	10.00	Autonomic balancer and sympathetic restorative.
Zanthoxylum clavaherculis fructus	5.00	Diffusive peripheral circulatory stimulant.
Dosage: 5 ml tid aq ac.	100.00	

Case history: leg ulceration

This lady, aged 66, presents with an ulceration on the ankle of her right leg, which she has had for a number of years. She previously had an ulcer on her left leg and she has had episodes of cellulitis. She also has rheumatoid arthritis and ulcerative colitis for which she is not seeking treatment.

Clinical signs:
Blood pressure: 170/85.
Pulse: 88.
Pulse pressure: 85.
CVI: 22,440.
Tongue: slight pale, swollen, slight anterior heat.

Analysis:
The pulse pressure and CVI suggest that this lady may have significant cardiovascular disease and she requires urgent assessment of possible diabetes. She has two major conditions of inflammation, and care must be taken to prevent emotional deconstruction, with potentially serious consequences. The formulation is aimed principally at reducing inflammation and tissue healing. Unfortunately, topical treatment was not possible because the ulcer was being medically treated.

Herb	Dosage	Actions
Achillea millefolium	15.00	Diffusive peripheral circulatory vasodilator. Anti-inflammatory. Tissue restorative.
Centella asiatica	15.00	CNS regulator and adaptogen. Anti-inflammatory and tissue healing.
Schizandra chinensis	10.00	Tonic adjunct and facilitator.
Hydrastis canadensis	15.00	Anti-inflammatory. Antiseptic, Alterative.
Symphytum officinale herba	15.00	Tissue healer and restorative. Foundational nutritional tonic.
Calendula officinale	15.00	Anti-inflammatory. Tissue healer.
Rosmarinus officinale	10.00	Autonomic balancer and sympathetic restorative.
Cinnamomum zeylanicum	5.00	Warming circulatory stimulant.
Dosage: 5 ml tid aq ac.	100.00	

The digestive system

The key to the diagnosis and treatment of digestive complaints is to distinguish whether it is essentially a functional disturbance or an organic condition.

Autonomic regulation

The condition of the GIT can only be understood in relation to the global working of the constitution as a whole and will reflect the balance of the ANS. Sympathetic activation will result in reduced visceral activity and hence reduced digestion system activity. Conversely, parasympathetic activation will result in increased visceral activity and hence increased digestive system activity. Sympathetic deficiency will result in a pattern similar to parasympathetic engagement. The main difference between sympathetic deficiency and parasympathetic excess is in the associated mood. Sympathetic deficiency is generally associated with low mood, lethargy and lack of motivation, whilst parasympathetic excess is generally associated with anxiety. Commonly there is a mixture of both patterns.

Sympathetic activity promotes gall bladder relaxation, parasympathetic promotes gall bladder secretion.

Sympathetic activation	Reduced intestinal motility. Reduced enzymatic secretion. Contraction of sphincters. Glycogenolysis. Reduces activity of the Brunner's glands.	Reduced appetite.

(Continued)

Parasympathetic activation	Increased intestinal motility. Increased enzymatic secretion. Relaxation of sphincters. Glycogenesis. Stimulates Brunner's glands.	Loose bowels or constipation. Wind and bloating. Low blood sugar. Increased appetite.

The fundamental energy status of the organism affects digestive system efficiency, both directly and through the induction of autonomic passive sympathetic deficiency. Age and depletion create deficiency of function and a tendency to visceroptosis, i.e. organ and tissue weakness creates hypotonicity, the organs weaken and tend to prolapse into the pelvic cavity. This is associated with changes in appetite and the volume of food capable of being digested effectively, the capacity to digest certain foods, e.g. salads, and general signs of weakened function; wind, bloating, indigestion, changes in bowel habit. All indications of SLUD.

Inflammation

Differentiate between inflammation, irritation and infection, or all three may be present. The digestive system may become a portal for the expression of inflammatory heat (as in Chinese medicine, liver heat invading the digestive tract.). This may be the explanation for inflammation where there is no clear cause, i.e. pathogenic infection. Heat would generally be expected to be evident from inspection of the tongue. Endogenous heat often tracks to the upper digestive tract producing symptoms such as heart burn and acid reflux, but is also a potential cause of inflammatory bowel disease. The resolution of such a manifestation requires emotional healing as part of the therapeutic intervention. The digestive herbs belonging to the Rose family are specific: Agrimonia, Potentilla erectum, Potentilla anserine, Geum, Filipendula.

Infection	Acute viral and bacterial. Chronic infection, e.g. fungal (candida). Bacterial (e.g. Helicobacter pylori). Parasites.
Allergy and food sensitivity Lectins	Commonly a complication of parasympathetic over activity.
Food qualities Cold food	(e.g. raw food, salad, ice cream, cold drinks, fruit) suppresses function, decreases digestive capability. Thymoleptic shock in acute cases. (e.g. alcohol, spices, meat) causes irritation.
Hot food	Congestion and heat.
Sweet food	Creates congestion.

(*Continued*)

Greasy food Dairy food	Has a 'sliding' action which is demulcent and antacid but creates mucus congestion.
Dietary protocols Eating patterns Food combinations	Irregular eating patterns, missing meals, eating when preoccupied or busy or stressed, excessive, or inadequate consumption. Difficult combinations for digestion, e.g. fats and carbohydrate. Protein and carbohydrate (e.g. The Hay Diet).
Nutritional deficiencies	May follow debilitating digestive conditions leading to malabsorption problems.
Mucus	Mucus is produced by hyper-functioning membranes related to increased parasympathetic tone, irritation, or food sensitivity. Catarrhal membranes may result in poor impaired digestion and nutrient absorption. Mucus created in the digestive tract will commonly be evident on the tongue.
Abdominal pain	The organ involved needs to be identified. In general, colicky pain related to food intake or bowel movement is intestinal in origin. IBS is a generic condition marked by vague to severe pain accompanied by wind, bloating and bowel disturbance, usually alternating constipation and looseness and is generally a related to changes in the ANS.
Disturbances of bowel function	Excessive looseness is different to diarrhoea and doesn't have the characteristic appearance and smell. It is a symptom of increased gut mobility rather than pathogenic invasion and can be very marked. Pathogenic infection has an incubation phase of 24 hours, symptoms of sickness and diarrhoea which follow within hours of ingestion of food is generally the consequence of the ingestion of bacterial toxins. Constipation may relate to hypertonicity or deficiency. Long term use of laxatives weakens the digestion.

Classification of herbs for physiological actions on the gastrointestinal system

Actions	Herbal intervention
Antacids	Filipendula ulmaria, Curcuma longa, Chamomilla spp. Hydrastis canadensis. Demulcents: Ulmus fulva, Aloe vera.
Antiemetics	Ballota nigra—general application (vestibular), pregnancy. Chamomilla spp., Mentha piperita, Zingiberis officinalis Nervines.
Stomachic Toning to the gastric membrane. Achlorhydria.	Geum urbana, Acorus calamus. Centaurium erythraea. Agrimonia, eupatorium. Angelica archangelica. Chamomilla spp.
General stimulants	Bitters—Gentiana lutea. Artemisia spp. Cichorium intybus. Centaurium erythraea. Marsdenia condurango. Chelone glabra.
Bowel stimulants	Aperients: Rheum off, Rumex crispus, Taraxacum officinale radix. Glycyrrhiza glabra. Linum usitatissimum. Laxatives: Rhamnus frangula, Rhamnus cathartica, Sambucus nigra (bark). Juglans cinera. Purgatives: Cassia angustifolia/acutifolia (Senna), Aloe spp.
Tonic hepatic/digestive For torpid conditions. Stimulating to the liver, gall bladder, pancreas and digestive tract—increasing secretions, improving absorption, cleansing and toning to catarrhal conditions of the digestive mucous membranes.	Berberis aquifolium, Berberis vulgaris, Collinsonia canadensis, Rheum officinalis, Rhamnus spp., Rumex, crispus. Leptandra Chionanthus virginicus. Chelone glabra.
Spasmolytics	Chamomilla recutita, Chamaemelum nobile, Dioscorea villosa, Mentha spp., Viburnum opulus, Valeriana, Lavendula. Solanaceous for acute spasm—Atropa belladonna, Hyoscyamnus niger.
Carminatives Relaxant, spasmolytic, stimulating, antiseptic, anti-inflammatory. Improve circulation to the tissues, anti-catarrhal, local action on the digestive reflexes.	Mentha spp., Chamomilla spp., Angelica archangelica. Melissa officinalis. Juniperis officinalis. Rosmarinus officinalis. Thymus, officinalis. Salvia spp. Brassica nigra. Allium cepa. Armoracia rusticana. Allium sativa. Cinnamomum spp. Zingiberis officinalis. Elletaria, cardamomum. Pimpinella anethum. Foeniculum, Anethum gaveolums, Eugenia caryophyllus.

(Continued)

Classification of herbs for physiological actions on the gastrointestinal system (Continued)

Actions	Herbal intervention
Hot and pungent herbs, many of which contain mustard oils are particularly effective for cold/damp mucous congestion. Warming, carminative actions.	
Demulcents	Althaea off. Symphytum radix., Linum usitassium. Glycyrrhiza glabra. Plantago spp., Cetraria islandica. Chondrus crispus. Ulnus fulva, Borago officinale.
Astringents Particularly useful for treating chronic catarrhal conditions and improving tissue tone and integrity. Used for the treatment of overactivity and diarrhoea. Balancing and integrating to central function.	Filipendula ulmaria, Hydrastis Canadensis. Geum urbanum, Agrimonia eupatorium. Potentilla erecta.
Anti-infectives May be specific to certain pathogens or general immune enhancing.	Baptisia tinctoria, Echinacea spp., Salvia spp., Hydrastis canadensis, Thymus officinalis. Origanum vulgare.
Tonics To improve vital energy of the system and immunological response. Essential in order to provide 'ground' for treatment. Generally, nourish, moisten and tissue healing.	Panax ginseng, Panax quinquifolium, Astragalus membranaceus. Atractylodes, Eleutherococcus senticosus. Codonopsis Rosmarinus officinalis.

Herbs for the digestive system

Herb	Therapeutic movement	Principal therapeutic actions
Acorus calamus	Stimulating, relaxing, decongesting, restoring.	Stimulating and relaxing digestive tonic with antispasmodic, pungent, bitter, sweet and cleansing action.
Alpinia officinarum	Resolving, decongesting, restoring. Stimulant, carminative.	Aromatic stimulant.
Chamomilla recutita	Relaxing, calming, decongesting. Bitter. Sweet. Moist.	Sedating and relaxing for conditions of overactivity. Anti-inflammatory. Releases congested heat, moistens and soothes.
Chicorium intybus	Bitter. Sweet. Salty. Cool. Moist.	Digestive tonic. Blood tonic. Hepatic, cholagogue. choleretic, splenic. Laxative. Antibacterial.
Filipendula ulmaria	Decongesting, astringing.	Astringent tonic to the gastrointestinal membranes. Diaphoretic. Anti-inflammatory. Silica content.
Gentiana lutea	Bitter. Astringent. Cold. Dry.	Bitter digestive tonic. Antiseptic, antibacterial Cholagogue. Hepatic. Emmenagogue.
Hydrastis canadensis	Restoring, stimulating, decongesting, transformative.	Astringent, anti-inflammatory, depurative, anti-infective tonic. Membrane restorative. Vasotonic. Cleansing action.

Conditions applicable and combinations	Energetic actions and notes
One of the best general tonics for deficient digestion—fatigue, diarrhoea, bloating, anorexia. Acute gastritis, hypo or hyperacidity. Gastrointestinal catarrh and congestion. Chronic ulcers, abscesses, skin eruptions. Deficient, congested digestive conditions associated with flatulence, fermentation and bloating.	
Tension, restlessness. Oversensitivity. Gastric and duodenal irritation and ulcers. Enteritis, IBS, deficient digestion. Dysmenorrhoea. Menopausal symptoms. PMS. Membrane irritation and inflammation.	Specific for digestive complaints in children.
Digestive deficiency and atony—anorexia, gastritis. Cholelithiasis. Liver and splenic obstructions Constipation. Rheumatism, gout. **Special features: digestive and hepatic tonic to improve digestive function, clears heat and toxicity from the blood, digestive tract and liver, and tonic for blood deficiency and general depletion and weakness.**	Specific for rising liver heat associated with false fire.
Hyperacidity associated with gastritis, ulceration, dyspepsia. Oesophageal burning. Diarrhoea and bowel disturbance. Dispersive, circulatory action in fevers or stagnation. Rheumatism, arthritis and gout. Chronic tissue weakness.	Soothing, reassuring and uplifting.
GIT deficiency. Gastric atony. Nausea. Flatulence/bloating. Hepatic and splenic. Tonic to the GIT, improving appetite and digestive efficiency. Improves the hepatic portal system, facilitating nutritional absorption. Facilitates conditions of energy depletion and exhaustion.	Intense bitter action with restoring, invigorating and discharging action.
Restorative for all membranes and digestive organs—gastritis, gastroenteritis, constipation, gall stones. Venous tonic—haemorrhage, fibroids, varicose veins, haemorrhoids. Uterine stimulant and astringent.	Intense resolving action.

(Continued)

Herb	Therapeutic movement	Principal therapeutic actions
Potentilla erecta	Restoring, resolving, stabilising. Astringent. Bitter. Sweet.	Astringent, anti-inflammatory, anti-infective, tonic action.
Rheum officinalis	Astringing, restoring. Bitter. Astringent. Cold. Dry.	A bitter, astringent, tonic for the liver and gastrointestinal membranes. Laxative. Anti-inflammatory. Antiviral. Antiparasitic.
Rosmarinus officinale	Stimulating, relaxing, restorative, resolving. Bitter. Pungent.	Stimulant, relaxing and balancing tonic with an affinity for the digestive tract. Cerebral-spinal stimulant and restorative, adrenal tonic.

Case history: digestive disturbance

This 33-year-old housewife presents with a persistent digestive upset, which she has had for some three years. She has been diagnosed as suffering from IBS by her GP. She has received a number of medicines, which she reports as not effective, however is not receiving any treatment at the present time. She has frank diarrhoea 6–7 times per normal day, which is accompanied by pain and blood and mucous on occasions. Her symptoms are worse in the mornings and eating precipitates diarrhoea. She is inclined to acid indigestion, wind and bloating. The diarrhoea is aggravated by most vegetables, particularly the brassicas, most fruit and any foods of a rough or angular texture. She is inclined to hypoglycaemia. She feels tired and 'nervy'. She feels the cold easily and is inclined to cold peripheral circulation. Her menstrual cycle is of normal length, flow and regularity.

Clinical signs:
Blood pressure: 120/84.
Pulse: 86.
Pulse pressure: 36.
CVI: 17,888.
Tongue: very pale base, superficial heat papillae to the tip, close white coating—thick at the rear, dry surface.

Abdominal examination: NAD apart from some general tenderness.

The patient is married with no children. She has an attractive, well-groomed appearance and is of normal weight. She appears nervous and hesitant. She describes herself as a worrier.

Conditions applicable and combinations	Energetic actions and notes
Haemorrhage, irritation, or infection of the gastrointestinal tract, acute or chronic diarrhoea. Digestive system deficiency—loose bowels, fatigue, prolapse.	Resolving action for congested heat patterns.
Deficient digestion—anorexia, indigestion, nausea. Hepatitis. Pancreatitis. Jaundice. Amenorrhea. Stimulates peristalsis in the large intestine and tones the digestive tract generally.	
Digestive deficiency conditions. Headache from deficiency. Circulatory weakness. Adaptogenic. Antiseptic and immune enhancing.	Principal ANS balancing herb.

Therapeutic analysis:

It is important to distinguish whether she is suffering from a functional disturbance or an organic disease. The presence of blood in the stools and the severity and chronicity of the disturbance suggests that this condition is or is at the start of an inflammatory bowel condition, in this case mucous colitis. There is a need to distinguish diarrhoea from loose bowels. The syndrome needs treating as well as the disharmony as this is potentially serious. There is a red flag for bowel cancer, which often follows protracted bowel dysfunction. She requires orthodox biomedical investigation.

The clinical signs suggest a hyper-parasympathetic dysfunction with accompanying visceral constriction and overactivity. This is most probably related to anxiety, or specifically to a persistent state of hyperarousal due to a feeling of vulnerability, insecurity and agitation. The systolic is on the low side compared to the diastolic, suggesting some deficient sympathetic tone. The high pulse rate suggests some adrenaline activation, despite a low sympathetic tone. The high pulse may also be a possible indicator for anaemia. The cardiovascular index is high, and again suggest an adrenergic stress response, but the pulse pressure is low, suggesting that although she is agitated her profile is one of lack of control and deficiency.

The hyperaemic membranes are sensitised and hyper-reactive to foods, both in terms of immunological sensitivity and mechanical irritation. The congested, irritated and catarrhal membranes are indicated by the coating on the tongue and the presence of mucus and blood in the stools.

The tongue also demonstrates deficiency and poor blood perfusion by its pale character. Because of the liver and pancreatic overactivity, she suffers from hypoglycaemia, which is a complication to the general situation, i.e. initiates a physiological stress response.

The possibility of malabsorption from prolonged digestive upset needs to be considered, in particular fat soluble vitamins. Anaemia is a strong possibility and requires investigation.

Contextual understanding:

The dysfunction could have arisen because her sense of 'safety' was compromised following a series of challenging life events and shocks. These include the death of her father following a long illness with cancer, several other deaths in the family, a car accident and a particularly difficult upset at a family party with a domineering elderly aunt. Her limbic brain now perceives her situation as being chronically perilous, which elicits a stress hormone response. The orientation determined by the ANS is one of internalisation of action. This is response is the outcome of an assessment by her limbic brain of experiential learning and resource capability. The transition of the problem from a functional digestive disturbance to an organic condition is a probably a combination of a deteriorating tissue state together with a further somatisation of the disharmony.

Medicine composition

Herb	Dosage	Action
Eleutherococcus senticosus	20.00	Endocrine tonic, adaptogen, CNS regulator.
Curcuma longa	10.00	Anti-inflammatory, antioxidant.
Chamomilla recutita	15.00	Relaxant, demulcent, anti-inflammatory.
Potentilla erectum	15.00	Astringent, relaxant, tissue tonic. Resolvent for endogenous heat.
Borago officinale	15.00	Adrenal restorative, tissue healer.
Althaea officinale radix	15.00	Demulcent, tissue healer.
Rosmarinus officinalis	15.00	ANS regulator, adaptogen, restorative.
Elletaria cardamomum	5.00	Aromatic, carminative.
Dosage: 5 ml of tincture to be given three or four times daily in a little water.	110.00	

Medicine rationale:

The medicine is designed to act directly on the physiological symptoms as well as the underlying disharmony so that there is an interconnection in resolution between levels, i.e. at the tissue and organ level and within the limbic brain and the control of the ANS. This ensures that there is a true resolution, which should be assessable in terms of behaviour and the personal sense of well-being of the patient.

The Eleutherococcus is to establish a solid energy foundation by tonification of the endocrine system, strengthening of the adrenal, liver and pancreatic function and establishment of regulation within the HPA axis. The consequence is a reduction in the stress response. Experientially, the patient develops a 'sense' of control and integrity and a 'feeling' of more personal control, stability and authority. The Rosmarinus is an additional aid to the regulation of the ANS, as well as providing additional endocrine support. It also promotes the movement of blood to the head and periphery, giving additional emphasis to the movement of the formula.

The Curcuma, Chamomilla, Potentilla, Borago and Althaea contribute their different actions to resolve inflammation, relax, astringe, soften and heal the mucous membranes and tissues at a physical level, and at an energetic level engender a feeling of release, reassurance, balance and regulation. The Elletaria lifts the tone of the formulae, assisting in the energetic movement and the resolution of negative emotional impressions.

One year:
Blood pressure: 105/68.
Pulse: 74.
Pulse pressure: 37.
Tongue: Pink base, slight dry coating to the rear.

Symptoms NAD. Some tolerance of fruit and vegetable intake. Feeling calmer and more energised.

Case history: digestive complaint

The patient is a 40-year-old therapist who complains of persistent digestive problems, which have been worsening over a period of five weeks. He has frequent, loose bowel movements, which are accompanied by spastic pain. There is occasional bright blood, but no mucus, and a feeling of tenesmus and bloating. The number of bowel movements reduced to three times daily when he became meticulous with his diet, i.e. avoiding wheat and daily products, abrasive foods, spices and alcohol. He has a dull pain in the upper right quadrant of his abdomen. He reports his energy as being very low. He feels the cold in the periphery and centre.

This man has a long history of digestive disorder, particularly acid indigestion and turbulence and bloating. He describes himself as having sensitivity to bread, white rice, mushrooms and dairy food. He also has a long history of problems with fatigue. He has recently been through a considerable amount of stress through financial and family problems although the situation has now improved.

Clinical signs:
Blood pressure: 90/70 (previous readings: 140/86, 110/70).
Pulse: 80.
Pulse pressure: 20.
Tongue: very pale and swollen with a loose white coating and a central fissure.

He has a sociable, outgoing personality, articulate and able to express his situation clearly and intelligently. He appears slightly dishevelled and is slightly overweight, particularly around the abdomen. He appears very pale to the point of greyness and has dark rings under his eyes. He works long hours as a self-employed therapist. He is married with one son aged 12.

Analysis:
The clinical signs clearly demonstrate a marked sympathetic deficiency within the ANS with the characteristic symptoms of fatigue, blood deficiency, cold patterning and internalised functioning, i.e. excessive overworking of the digestive system. The blood and tenesmus are concerning and possibly indicative of organic disease, cancer or inflammatory bowel disease. The man has three instances of bowel cancer within his family, including his father, and he requires immediate further investigation.

Herb	Dosage	Actions
Angelica sinensis	15.00	Optimising the movement of blood and blood tonic.
Codonopsis	20.00	Foundational energy.
Astagalus membraneous	20.00	Immunological support and tonification.
Schizandra chinensis	10.00	Adjuncts for tonification. Movement of the fire principal.
Taraxacum officinald radix	20.00	Liver support and tonification. Emotional support.
Glycyrrhiza glabra	15.00	Nourishing tonic. Tissue depurative.
Rosmarinus officinalis	15.00	Balancing of the ANS.
Borago officinale	20.00	Adrenal support. Support with courage and resolution.
Potentilla erectum	15.00	Digestive regulator. Resolvent for endogenous heat.
Dosage: 5 ml tid aq ac.	150.00	

Rationale:
To provide tonic support for his foundational energy and immunological support and to balance the ANS system and digestive system, whilst medical investigation is in progress.

Four weeks:
Blood pressure: 120/75.
Pulse: 72.
Pulse pressure: 45.

Energy improved. Some improvement in digestive symptoms—reduced bloating, reduced pain, no blood in the stools, stool constituency improved. Bowel cancer is confirmed and he is waiting for surgery.

Case history: indigestion

This retired gardener, aged 65, complains of stomach ache, which has been worsening over a period of several weeks. The main symptom is a burning indigestion pain felt under the ribs. His bowels are normally regular and well formed, but have recently been looser. He frequently has wind following ingestion of food and his digestion is generally uncomfortable.

He complains of feeling tired, particularly in the evenings, and generally feels better with activity. He has frequent dull, muzzy headaches. His extremities are generally cold. He has generalised muscular aches and pains. He has nocturia up to four times per night and investigations revealed some prostate enlargement. Cystoscopy is normal.

This gentleman is well nourished, of normal weight and appears sprightly but looks slightly older than his 65 years. He worked as a manager of a manufacturing firm until redundancy, five years ago, when he became self-employed as a gardener. He has a large garden of his own where he spends much of his time looking after and growing vegetables.

Investigations:
Blood tests for anaemia and B12 are negative.

Clinical signs:
Blood pressure: 144/80.
Pulse: 60.
Pulse pressure: 64.
Tongue: moderate colour, slightly swollen, slight heat in the tip.

Analysis:
A judgement needs to be made as to whether this patient is suffering from a specific identifiable biomedical condition, such as gastritis, peptic ulcer, oesophageal reflux or a more generalised digestive disturbance significant upon a constitutional dysfunction. An organic condition or syndrome would call for priority of treatment.

He has indications of endocrine depletion, i.e. his energy is reported as poor and his energy recovery is poor, such that a heavy day's work has a repercussion for the next day. He has indications of deficiency, despite a relatively high sympathetic activation, as denoted by the relatively high systolic blood pressure. His extremities tend to be cold; he has cerebral circulatory deficiency and his visceral processes are hyper-functional. The blood pressure may indicate significant cardiovascular disease. This could relate to diabetic changes affecting sugar irregularities. The adrenal, liver, pancreatic axis is of considerable importance, irrespective of the diabetes issue, as it is the foundation of the central energy.

The digestive symptoms are most likely due to a generalised increase in parasympathetic activity, this manifests as an increase in digestive function, i.e. increased acid secretions, loose bowels, wind and bloating and also increased urinary tract activity. The parasympathetic activity is over-functioning in relationship to the sympathetic activity and accounts for the net sympathetic deficiency.

Composition

Herb	Dosage	Actions
Panax ginseng	20.00	Endocrine tonic, adaptogen, ANS and CNS balancer.
Astragalus membraneous	15.00	Endocrine tonic, adaptogen, immune regulator.
Curcuma longa	10.00	Antioxidant, hepato protector.
Leptandra decantra	10.00	Liver stimulant, drainer.

(Continued)

Composition (Continued)

Herb	Dosage	Actions
Carduus marianus	15.00	Liver restorative and protector.
Symphytum officinale radix	15.00	Endocrine restorative, liver restorative.
Rosmarinus officinalis	10.00	ANS balancer, digestive regulator.
Elletaria cardamomum	5.00	Aromatic, carminative.
Filipendula ulmaria	10.00	Aromatic disperser, decongestant, antacid.
	110.00	

The key to the intervention is a restorative, decongesting action to the core organs of the liver, pancreas and endocrine systems. Panax, Astragalus and Schizandra are an integral combination aimed at sympathetic restoration, endocrine tonification and the associated 'sense of' balance and power.

The Curcuma, Carduus, Leptandra and Symphytum have a draining and restorative action on the liver and pancreas. Rosmarinus is a general regulator and also specific for digestive regulation. Elletaria and Filipendula are aromatic dispersers to enhance function, lift emotional tone and move the formula. The Filipendula, Elletaria, Curcuma and Symphytum in particular also have symptomatic effects directly on the digestive symptoms through demulcent, antacid, astringent and carminative actions.

Three weeks:
Blood pressure: 130/76.
Tongue: reduced heat.

General improvement in energy and well-being. Digestion symptom-free for two weeks.

The liver

The liver is the key central physiological processor to regulate, convert and transform all substances ingested. Similarly, energetically the liver is the seat of the function to regulate, synthesise, integrate and transmute the energetic function of the body, in particular emotional impressions.

Autonomic regulation

The liver acts as one of the primary blood reservoirs and so internalisation of blood movement from a net autonomic sympathetic deficiency will inevitably cause blood retention in the liver and potentially liver congestion. Psychogenic factors will cause deficiency through active sympathetic deficiency and parasympathetic excess. Fatigue factors will cause passive sympathetic deficiency, i.e. tiredness creates stagnation of blood movement and hence visceral congestion.

Sources of disharmony

Infection	Hepatitis A, B, C, D and E leptospirosis or Weil's disease. Epstein-Bar cytomegalovirus.	
Dietary	Fatty foods. Food allergy and sensitivity. Alcohol and drugs.	Particularly 'masked' food allergy inducing a stress hormone reaction. Note racial and cultural variations of exposure. Often difficult to eliminate.

(Continued)

	Food additives, e.g. MSG. Poisons and toxins. Herb–drug interactions.	Cytochrome P_{45}, e.g. CYP3A system inducted by Hypericum. Cytochrome P_{445} inducted by nicotine. Inhibition of metabolic enzymes by herbs and foods, e.g. flavonoids, polycyclic aromatic hydrocarbons.
Obstruction	Cholelithiasis. Cholangitis. Carcinoma—common bile duct.	

Courvoisier's law

States that in the presence of a palpable gall bladder, jaundice is unlikely to be caused by gall stones. This is because gall stones are formed over a long period of time and this results in a shrunken, fibrotic gall bladder, which does not distend easily. Therefore, the gall bladder is more often enlarged in pathologies that cause obstruction of the biliary tree, which occur over a shorter period of time, such as pancreatic malignancy, than in gallstone disease.

Inflammation

As liver congestion is the consequence of autonomic dysregulation and internalised blood dynamics it follows that the liver will be the seat of the internalised emotion associated with it. Liver heat may be complicated by alcohol and drug use taken to control repressed emotion and by food intolerances and poor diet and nutrition. However, non-alcohol related fatty liver disease can be present in situations of good lifestyle, diet and nutrition and in this situation is attributable to liver congestion due to autonomic dysregulation. The liver is associated, at least functionally, with anger and assertion. 'Rising liver heat' may characteristically be expressed through the manifestation of heat in the throat, e.g. chronic sore throat, recurrent tonsillitis and in the longer term, thyroiditis. 'False fire' is a term used to denote emotional expression that is a corruption of the manifestation of assertion, e.g. irritability, passive-aggressive behaviour, destructive criticism.

Relationship to other organ systems

- Energy status—links with adrenal glands.
- Hormone systems:
  - Hormone deficiency can lead to liver disharmony.
  - Liver stagnation may lead to hormone deficiency through nutritional factors and actions on the ANS.
- The functions of the liver and pancreas are intimately related and herb actions are essentially the same for both.

- Liver function can have significant effect on other organ systems, e.g. blood dynamics and the reproductive system. SHBG (sex hormone binding globulin) removes excess oestrogen.

The control of liver physiology

The liver is regarded as functionally connected with the gall bladder and pancreas, and as a blood reservoir with the spleen.

The liver is influenced by the ANS through the regulation of the gall bladder in relation to digestive function. Sympathetic action causes relaxation of the gall bladder, a decrease in bile production and an increase in glycogenolysis resulting in a net reduction in liver activity. Parasympathetic action causes contraction of the gall bladder, an increase in bile production and an increase in glycogenesis. The liver is extremely liable to influence from the overall balance of the ANS through its function as a blood reservoir. High sympathetic tone reduces blood volume in the liver through increasing blood flow to the muscular-skeletal system and the brain, whilst low sympathetic tone and high parasympathetic tone increases the liver blood volume, which if persistent can result in blood stagnation in the liver. The opposite is also true, if the liver is involved in additional activity, for example in the detoxification of alcohol or toxins, fighting infection as in hepatitis or in IgG activity as a result of allergic processes, then there will be a concentration of activity and hence blood will be held in the liver. The key to control of liver function is the balance of the circulatory dynamics.

Summary of physiological mechanisms that affect the liver:

- Blood dynamics, i.e. ANS control of blood distribution
- The hepatic flow—the stimulation of bile movement by the action of the gall bladder
- The constriction of blood vessels and ducts within the hepatic system
- Hepatocellular integrity

It is essential to assess the level of liver involvement in a syndrome, i.e. whether a functional disturbance or parenchymal, and the therapeutic intervention can be directed accordingly.

Therapeutic intervention

Improving assertion, sense of control and good decision-making and releasing patterns of constraint and associated emotional disharmony.

Externalisation of blood and energy.	ANS regulation. Sympathetic restoratives parasympathetic drainers. Hepatic regulation.
Stimulate the hepatic flow.	Bitters. Hepatics.
Relax the liver circulation.	Relaxants.
Restore hepatocellular integrity.	Liver tropho-restoratives.

Classifications of herbal actions

Actions	Herbs
Cholagogues	Bitters. Centaurium erythraea. Chelidonium majua. Peumus boldus. Leptandra decandra Chionanthus virginicus. Berberis vulgaris, Rumex crispus. Chelone glabra. Fumaria officinalia.
Hepatoprotectives and restoratives	Carduus marianus, Carbenia benedictus, Cynara scolymus. Bupleurum. Taraxacum officinalis Radix. Schizandra chinensis. Lycium barbarum. Paeonia laterifolia. Curcuma longa. Glycyrrhiza spp. Polygonum multiflorum, Hypericum perforatom. Agropyron repens.
Rising liver heat syndrome Associated emotional resolution	Chicorium intybus, Centaurium erythraea. Hyssopus officinalia. Salvia officinalia. Marrubium vulgare. Iris versicolor. Rosa damascene. Agrimonia eupatorium.

Herbs for liver function

Herb	Therapeutic movement	Principal therapeutic actions
Agrimonia eupatorium	Harmonising. Balancing.	Astringent tonic for the liver and GIT.
Arctium lappa	Cleansing. Restorative. Harmonising. Soothing.	Wide acting depurative. Trophorestorative for the liver and kidneys.
Artemisia absinthium	Stimulating. Discharging.	Intense, stimulating, bitter, astringing, hepatic.
Berberis aquifolium	See below.	See below.

Actions	Herbs
Circulatory balance	Achillea millefolium. Angelica archangelica. Anemone pulsatilla.
Liver relaxants	Chrysanthemum vulgare. Paeonia laterifolia. Dioscorea villosa. Viburnum opulus, Leonorus cardiacca.
Liver Balance To restore inner and outer balance	Stachys betonica. Carbenia benedictus. Schizandra chinensis.
Hepatic portal circulation	Bitters. Hepatics. Collinsonia. Canadensis.
Digestive tonics	Chelone glabra. Marsdenia, Centaurium erythaea. Chicorium intybus. Leptandra decandra. Chionanthus virginicus. Gentiana lutea.
Anti-infectives	Hypericum perforatum. Thuja occidentalis. Echinacea angustifolia. Artemisa spp. Baptisia tinctoria. Hydrastis canadensis. Berberis vulgaris, Carbenia benedictus.

Conditions applicable and combinations	Energetic actions and notes
Clears toxic heat and congestion of membranes and promotes assimilation of nutrients.	Promotes the integration and assimilation of emotional tension associated with the liver and GIT.
Specific for rising toxic heat reactions especially affecting the head-acne, eczema, furunculosis.	Integrative and restorative. Root, seed and herb have different actions.
Stimulant for the liver, GB, GIT, kidneys, genitourinary tract (GUT) to increase function, discharge toxicity, promote immunity and resolve pathogenic infection and tumours. Neurasthenia with toxic heat.	Clearing chronic, deep, toxic, congested conditions. Combine with dispersing herbs and aromatics.
Liver stimulant and depurative specific for toxic heat conditions especially associated with skin complaints.	

(Continued)

Herb	Therapeutic movement	Principal therapeutic actions
Berberis vulgaris	Opening. Discharging.	Stimulating and relaxing hepatic. Stimulant for the digestive processes. Membrane tonic and cleanser. Bowel tonic and stimulant.
Carduus marianus	Restoring. Nutritive.	Hepatoprotective and regenerative at the tissue level.
Carbenia benedictus	Restoring. Decongesting. Harmonising.	Combined actions of stimulating and restorative hepatic with diaphoresis.
Chelidonium majus	Discharging. Draining. Releasing.	Bitter, stimulant for the liver, gall bladder and pancreas. Spasmolytic for the gall ducts.
Chelone glabra		Gentle stimulant for the liver and GIT.
Chionanthus virginica	Stimulating. Invigorating.	Stimulating and relaxing hepatic. Promotes biliary and pancreatic secretions.
Cynara scolymus	Restorative, balancing, harmonising. Salty.	Restorative and regenerative for the liver and kidneys.
Dioscorea villosa	Relaxing. Resolving.	Autonomic nerve relaxant for the liver and GIT. GIT and GB spasm and irritation.
Euonymus atropurp.	Stimulating. Invigorating.	Stimulating and relaxing hepatic and digestive.
Fumaria officinalis	Stimulating. Relaxing.	Stimulant and antispasmodic for the liver and GB.
Gentiana lutea	Discharging. Restorative.	Stimulating, intensely bitter restorative for liver and GIT function.

Conditions applicable and combinations	Energetic actions and notes
Stimulant for torpid, catarrhal and congested conditions of the liver, gall bladder and digestive tract.	
Acute toxicity. Hepatitis.	Restorative.
Headache and cerebrospinal circulatory deficiency related to congestion, deficiency and toxicity of the liver and GIT. ANS balancer through hepatic regulation.	Emotional balancer, gives sense of harmony and perspective.
Cholelithiasis with acute spasm. Spastic constipation. Combine with carminatives and relaxants.	Combine with carminatives and relaxants. Schedule 3, low dosages.
Atonic, debilitated conditions of the liver, pancreas and GIT to improve appetite and function for children and the infirm.	
Atonic, congested conditions of the liver, gall bladder, pancreas to improve tone and function. Carbohydrate metabolism and blood sugar regulation.	
Tissue restorative and balancer.	
Neuralgia. Rheumatic syndromes related to the hepatic and digestive dysfunction. Especially syndromes related to hormone deficiency. Dysmenorrhoea.	Pituitary balancing.
Torpid conditions with deficiency, congestion associated with digestive dysfunction, anorexia, constipation and hepatic stasis.	
Skin conditions particular associated with liver heat congestion—eczema, psoriasis.	
Torpid, deficient and debilitated states to improve appetite, digestive function and absorption. Hepatoportal congestion.	Harmonises the internal equilibrium. Small doses. Combine with modifying agents and aromatics.

(Continued)

Herb	Therapeutic movement	Principal therapeutic actions
Glycyrrhiza glabra/ uralensis (prepared and raw)	Relaxing. Restoring.	Restoring and regulating for endocrine system (adrenals, pituitary, gonads) and the liver and pancreas. Anti-infective, immune enhancing and stimulating.
Hydrastis canadensis	Resolving. Transforming. Harmonising. Stimulating.	Stimulating, relaxing and astringent tonic for the liver, pancreas, GIT and membranes. Anti-infective. Haemostatic and coagulant.
Iris versicolor	Resolving. Discharging.	Stimulating alterative for chronic congestion of the liver, GB, lymphatics and intestinal glands. Hepatic congestion resultant on venous or lymphatic congestion.
Leptandra decandra	Stimulant. Discharging.	Stimulating and relaxing hepatic and GIT agent.
Lycium barbarum	Restoring. Harmonising.	Restorative for the liver and kidneys. Adaptogenic.
Marrubium vulgare	Stimulating. Draining.	Stimulating bitter and resolvent for the liver and kidneys.
Paeonia spp.	Relaxing and restorative for the liver and pancreas.	Transformative agent for hepatic congestion with toxic heat and deficiency. Hepatorestorative.
Schizandra chinensis	Dispersing. Harmonising. Discharging.	Hepatoprotective and restorative for the liver. Clears liver toxicity and heat. Adaptogenic.
Taraxacum officinalis radix	Resolving. Dissolving. Reassuring. Connecting.	Cleansing, harmonising and relaxing tonic and restorative for the liver, GB, pancreas, GIT and kidneys for both deficiency and excess conditions.

Conditions applicable and combinations	Energetic actions and notes
All conditions of inflammation, irritability, hypersensitivity. Protective and restorative action for liver toxicity and heat patterns.	
Resolves chronic conditions of irritation, inflammation, congestion and heat of the membranes of all systems. Chronic blood stasis of the liver, spleen, GIT, uterus. Hepatoportal congestion. Rising heat.	Agent for transformation. 'The' remedy for congestion. Low dose. Avoid in pregnancy.
Chronic rheumatic syndromes, herpes, eczema and psoriasis consequent upon toxic hepatic heat and congestion particularly rising heat issues (throat, head). Enlarged thyroid. Fibroids. Congestion and carcinoma of the breasts.	Promotes personal expression and stimulates creativity.
Torpid and congestive conditions of the liver, GB and GIT.	
Specific for eye conditions related to liver dysfunction. Tissue dryness associated with liver function.	
Rising heat conditions associated with the lungs and throat. Chronic torpid conditions—obesity, toxaemia, stagnation.	
Relaxant affect specific for liver congestion related to hormonal irregularities. Resolves emotional tension associated with liver dysfunction.	Tradition in Chinese medicine for beautifying the skin.
Specific for regulating the 'fire energy' for patterns of false fire (neck, shoulder tension, headache etc). ANS balancer and regulator.	With Carduus, Taraxacum, Glycyrrhiza.
Hepatic heat and congestion—eczema, acne, herpes. Restorative action for the liver, pancreas, adrenals, kidneys and connective tissues. Specific for deep muscular tension.	Releases deep patterns of emotional tension especially associated with the liver. Establishes balance and reassurance.

Case history: hepatitis

This 42-year-old lady presents with persistent abdominal pain, tenderness and bloating, which she has had for three or four days. She is queasy and anorexic. She experiences alternating hot and cold and feels prickly. She feels tired and lethargic. Her general health is reported as normally very good. There is some history of IBS with an inclination to constipation.

She is of an attractive, well dressed and well-groomed appearance and of a sociable and articulate disposition. Weight is normal. She describes herself as physically very fit and active and is a regular dancer.

Clinical signs:
Blood pressure: 120/75.
Pulse pressure: 45.
Pulse: 84.
Tongue: slightly pale and swollen. Close white coating.

Blood results

	1 month	2 months	3 months	1 year	6 years	Reference range
Bilirubin	145	236	41		13	2–20
AST	2,857	1,156	164	48	37	29	7–55
ALT	3,454	1,254	211	29	27	31	8–48
Alk. Phosp	474	440	250	127	114	140	<250
Protein	71		72	68	74	56–85
Albumin	40		44	43	46	35–52
GGT			48	18	24	<40

The blood test shows significant hepatocellular damage and subsequently the patient was diagnosed with hepatitis B. The symptoms, although significant of some degree of infection, are not proportionate to the degree of seriousness of the problem. There was no presentation of jaundice, although as evidenced by the blood results, there was some disturbance of conjugation of bilirubin, however, this was not very significant.

The clinical signs show a pattern of slight constraint and slight deficiency, which is consistent with the tongue pattern of pale and swollen with catarrhal congestion. The pulse rate is elevated and suggests possibly a slight pyrexia. The treatment pattern is aimed primarily at hepatocellular restoration.

There is a need for significant protective and restorative action at the cellular level, prescribed in material dosage. In this case, this was implemented using Carduus marianus fresh juice. Other options could have been Curcuma powder, Taraxacum radix (decoction or juice), Cynara (juice or herb infusion), Agropyron (decoction).

Herbal tincture formulation

Herb	Dosage	Actions
Achillea Millefolium	15.00	Circulatory facilitator.
Centella asiatica	15.00	ANS and CNS balancer. Anti-inflammatory.
Eleutherococcus senticosis	20.00	Foundational tonic.
Schizandra chinensis	10.00	Tonic adjunct and the movement of fire.
Lycium barbarum	15.00	Hepatocellular restorative and aromatic.
Hydrastis canadensis	15.00	Bitter liver drainer. Anti-infective.
Taraxacum radix	30.00	Hepatic restorative and tonic.
Agropyron repens	30.00	Hepatic restorative and tonic.
Cinnamon	5.00	Aromatic.
Dosage: 5 ml qid.	155.00	

Case history: hepatitis A

A 54-year-old single business man presents with increasing jaundice over a period of two weeks. He is extremely lethargic, hot and sweaty, has a dull pain in his upper right abdominal quadrant and is experiencing anorexia. He has been under considerable work stress over the past five years and has been working very long hours, he had just returned from a two week holiday in Italy. Previous health has been good with no significant previous medical conditions.

Clinical signs:
Blood pressure: 130/95.
Pulse: 88.
Pulse pressure: 35.

Abdominal examination reveals a tender liver detectable 2 cm below the right costal margin but with no further abnormalities. He is moderately obese.

Analysis:
The patient contracted hepatitis A whilst on holiday. His clinical signs show significant diastolic blood pressure constraint, which will significantly affect hepatic congestion and the recovery of the condition. This is therefore a priority for treatment in addition to liver restoratives.

Herb	Dosage	Actions
Achillea millefolium	15.00	Circulatory diffusive. Liver stimulant and restorative.
Centella asiatica	15.00	CNS and ANS balancer. Anti-infective. Anti-inflammatory.
Smilax officinalis	20.00	Foundation tonic. Detoxicant and anti-inflammatory.
Schizandra chinensis	15.00	Adjunct for tonification, movement of fire.

(Continued)

Herb	Dosage	Actions
Carduus marianus	20.00	Bitter liver tonic and cholagogue. Antiviral. Hepatocellular restorative.
Agropyron repens	20.00	Liver tonic and restorative.
Cinnamon zeylanicum	5.00	Aromatic and dispersive agent.
Dosage: 5 ml qid.	105.00	

Case history: liver congestion

A 32 year old male landscape contractor complains of extreme fatigue and anorexia following an acute sore throat two weeks previously. He contracted the sore throat a few days after finishing work for the Christmas holidays and this has now virtually disappeared leaving him with a dry and irritable cough. He is extremely fatigued and has been unable to eat anything substantial for the past two weeks, the thought of food makes him queasy but he has no vomiting. He feels prickly cold and has hot sweaty legs. His normal energy he describes as very good.

Clinical signs:
Blood pressure: 100/75.
Pulse: 52.
Pulse pressure: 25.

He has a tender, palpable liver and tenderness over the pancreas. This man is of normal weight and average height and not as muscular as his occupation might suggest. He is sociable, articulate and quietly spoken. He works for landscape contractors, usually working very long hours doing demanding physical work, away from home during the week. It is usual for the contract team to spend their evenings drinking in a local pub. He spends a considerable amount per week on alcohol. His father has recently been admitted to hospital suffering from alcohol induced pancreatitis. He is in a long-term committed relationship and has no children.

Analysis:
This patient has a complex combination of issues. His clinical signs indicate a significant degree of deficiency, which would be understandable following the cessation of a very physically demanding job for the holidays and demonstrates a considerable fatigue syndrome. The deficiency would have a significant implication for his immune system and he developed acute laryngotracheobronchitis, presumably from which he is still recovering. The deficiency state will impact significantly on congestion of the liver and pancreas. There is also the possibility of occupational contact with noxious chemicals and infection, e.g. leptospirosis, hepatitis, Epstein Barr.

Herb	Dosage	Actions
Angelica archangelica radix	10.00	Aromatic dispersive for the circulation.
Centella asiatica	10.00	CNS and ANS regulator. Tonic and adaptogen.
Panax ginseng	15.00	Foundational and endocrine tonic and adaptogen.
Schizandra chinensis	12.50	Liver tonic and disperser of heat.
Carduus marianus	20.00	Hepatocellular restorative.
Paeonia laterifoloia	12.50	Liver restorative and vascular relaxant.
Glycyrrhiza glabra	15.00	Liver and adrenal supportive.
Rosmarinus officinalis	10.00	ANS balancer.
Citrus limonum	5.00	Aromatic.
Dosage: 5 ml tid.	110.00	

The respiratory system

Autonomic regulation

Sympathetic activation (β2 receptor) causes bronchodilation, parasympathetic activation causes vasoconstriction.

Dyspnoea	Functional	Active	Sympathetic deficiency. Reaction to shock. Tightness in the lungs. Spasticity and wheezing.
		Passive	Sympathetic deficiency. Fatigue reducing the lung 'energy'. Feeling of heaviness and restraint.
	Obstruction	Passive	Tissue degeneration. Fibrosis. Fluid (cardiac function).
		Passive/active	COPD.
	Wheezing	Active	Parasympathetic activation/sympathetic deficiency Acute and chronic asthma.
	Irritable lung	Active	Parasympathetic activation/sympathetic deficiency. Membrane irritability and immunological activation.

Inflammation

The respiratory system is a primary route of the expression of inflammatory or endogenous heat. Heat tracks to the throat or the lungs and is the seat of an inflammatory process not directly related to pathogenic infection. In Chinese medicine this is called 'liver heat' invading the lungs. In the lungs it is often manifest as a characteristic strident 'barking' cough, which is non-productive and either unrelated to a pathogenic infection or follows on from it. In this situation the treatment intervention requires emotional resolution and a specific herbal intervention. The emotion primarily associated with the lungs is said to be grief.

Coughing and phlegm

Expectoration

Expectoration refers to the ability of the system to generate a productive cough and expel mucus from the system. It is dependent upon the condition of the mucous membrane secretion and vital response. The suppression of a cough is only acceptable under certain conditions (e.g. nervous generated coughs) and the aim of treatment is to ensure efficient expectoration.

Phlegm

Catarrh is generally a response to irritation, inflammation or infection as a protective mechanism. The origin of the catarrhal irritation may not necessarily be in the respiratory system, as the mucous membranes are continuous and will produce reflex reactions in other organs. Typically, food substances that create irritation in the upper digestive system cause phlegm in the respiratory system. Dairy food is a common aggravating factor.

Infection is typified by an acute, hot, inflamed membrane reaction, which eases upon the production of mucus and which may leave residual chronic catarrh. Catarrh is not an indication of infection but may be a predisposing factor, i.e. congestion or dampness. It may be yellow coloured where affected by heat or green if purulent with infection. Phlegm is usually associated with congestion of the mucous membranes and associated tissues, due to either local issues and/or autonomic dysregulation.

Pathogenic	Viral, bacterial, fungal.
Environmental	Elemental influences: cold, damp, heat, dryness.
	Allergens: pollens, spores.
	Irritant: smoke, fog, dust.
Dietary	Food intolerance and allergy.
	Irritants: dairy, greasy food.
	Nutritional deficiencies.

Therapeutic intervention

Analysis and interpretation of the clinical signs and symptoms will determine the underlying syndrome. Deficiency will require tonification and pectorals, spasticity will require spasmolytics, heat patterns will require resolution. Prunus serorinta is a member of the Rose family specific for the resolution of heat. Marrubium vulgare is specific for the invasion of heat from liver to lung.

Classification of herb physiological actions

Differentiate between herbs with physiological actions and herbs with psycho-physiological actions, i.e. the level of intervention.

Stimulating expectorants	
Generally, work through a stimulating/irritating action upon the upper digestive tract, which creates a reflex action in the respiratory system.	Lobelia inflata, Primula veris radix. Little used; Cephaelis (Ipecacuanha), Urginea (Squills), Bellis perenis, Polygala senega.
The presence of saponins is often significant, e.g. Saponaria.	
Aromatic pectorals	
Aromatics are reassuring and lifting, they assist the movement of function and mitigate against disharmony and shock.	Thymus, Hyssopus, Inula, Nepeta hederacea.
This category includes herbs with a significant volatile oil content.	Mustard, Onion, Armoracia, Allium sativa.
The oils are excreted through the lungs exerting a local action which may be antiseptic, anti-inflammatory, relaxant, stimulating to the circulation and anti-catarrhal.	Cinnamomum, Zingiberis, Elletaria, Pimpinella, Foeniculum, Angelica.
Hot and pungent herbs, many of which contain mustard oils, are particularly effective for cold/damp mucous congestion.	
Warming, stimulating and relaxing aromatics are often used for the same purpose within formulae.	
Anti-tussives	
Only applicable where the cough is non-functional.	Prunus serotina, Lactuca.
Spasmolytics	
Have an action to relax smooth muscle and are applicable to conditions where constriction is a major component, e.g. asthma.	Lobelia, Thymus, Hyssopus, Grindelia camporum, Euphorbia hirta, Inula.
The control of acute asthma is now seldom appropriate as a result of inhalers. Solanaceous herbs are particularly applicable for acute control.	Datura stromonium, Atropa belladonna.
Demulcents	
Contain polysaccharides, which have a similar constituency and action to mucous, reducing irritation and inflammation.	Althaea, Symphytum radix., Linum, Glycyrrhiza, Plantago spp, Cetraria, Tussilago, Verbascum, Pulmonaria, Borago, Drosera rotundifolia.
The action may be reflex through effects of the digestive tract.	
Their use may need modifying, i.e. demulcents are cool and moist and may not suit the 'ground' of some respiratory conditions.	
Emotionally, demulcents are nourishing, reassuring and cool 'fire'.	

(Continued)

Diaphoretics

Have important applications in the treatment of fevers to reduce pyrexia when dangerous.

Improve the ANS profile and immunological reactions of the body.

Move conditions and syndromes in an upward and outward.

Achillea, Sambucus, Eupatorium, Nepata cataria.

Astringents

Particularly useful for treating chronic catarrhal conditions and improving tissue tone and integrity.

Dispel tension and inflammation with associated emotional disharmony at the tissue level.

Euphrasia officinalis, Nepeta hederacea, Hydrastis canadensis, Verbascum thapsus, Solidago virgaurea.

Anti-allergics

A symptomatic action, which is sometimes applicable in acute allergic reactions.

Requires the administration of spasmolytics, anti-inflammatory, astringents, demulcents.

Ephedra sinica, Urtica dioica.

Anti-infectives

May be specific to certain pathogens or general immune enhancing, however treatment of infection is usually best dealt with, and should always be accompanied by, constitutional correction.

Baptisia tinctoria, Echinacea spp., Salvia spp., Hydrastis canadensis, Thymus, Inula.

Respiratory tonics

To improve the vital energy of the system, promote harmony and activate the immunological response.

Generally, nourish, moisten and heal tissue.

Should be used to underpin the vitality in most treatment regimens.

Caution with the use of tonics in presence of infection.

Panax ginseng, Panax quinquifolium, Astragalus, Withania, Hydrocotyl, Inula, Verbascum, Equisetum, Borago, Symphytum.

Herbs for the respiratory system

Herb	Therapeutic movement	Principal therapeutic actions	Conditions applicable and combinations	Energetic actions and notes
Asclepias tuberosa	Stimulating, relaxing, decongesting. Pungent. Cool. Bitter.	Stimulant, expectorant, antispasmodic and anti-inflammatory. Diaphoretic.	Hard, dry coughs. Croup. Bronchitis. Asthma. Pleurisy. Pneumonia. Promotes and restores gastrointestinal, liver and kidney function.	Sympathetic restorative action.
Euphorbia pilufiera		Bronchial relaxant.		

(Continued)

Herb	Therapeutic movement	Principal therapeutic actions	Conditions applicable and combinations	Energetic actions and notes
Euphrasia officinalis	Resolving, decongesting, restoring. Astringent. Bitter. Pungent. Cool.	Astringent and mildly stimulating tonic for the mucous membranes.	Upper respiratory and upper digestive irritation, inflammation and catarrh—rhinitis, hay fever, sinusitis, gastroenteritis. Affinity for the eyes—choroiditis, blepharitis, corneal opacity, poor eyesight. Mildly stimulating, cleansing and restorative for the kidneys and bladder. Mildly stimulating, bitter, restorative for the gastrointestinal system.	
Glechoma hederacea	Resolvent, restorative. Astringent. Aromatic.	Tonic, anti-catarrhal, expectorant and astringent for the upper respiratory and digestive systems. Aromatic.	Nasal and bronchial catarrh, sinusitis. Otitis media and related catarrh tinnitus and deafness. Deficient digestion.	Aromatic.
Inula helenium	Restoring, stimulating, decongesting. Bitter. Pungent. Warm.	Warming, stimulating, balancing and restoring tonic for chronic deficiency and fatigue. Enhances immune potential. Stimulating, warming, relaxing and antiseptic for cold, damp and deficient lung and gastrointestinal conditions.	Fatigue, debility, immune deficiency with tendency to infections. Chronic bronchitis, asthma, chronic parenchymal lung disorders. Infections of the lungs, bladder and urinary tract. Toxic conditions such as eczema.	Potential as a major herb for the treatment of immunological deficiency and autoimmunity. Has pituitary action, i.e. acts on the higher autonomic centres.

(Continued)

Herb	Therapeutic movement	Principal therapeutic actions	Conditions applicable and combinations	Energetic actions and notes
			Promotes oestrogen and progesterone insufficiency and hence menstrual deficiency.	
Lobelia inflata	Stimulating, relaxing and restoring. Bitter. Pungent. Warm.	Stimulant, relaxant and diffuse action with amphoteric action on the ANS to stimulate or relax sympathetic tone. Diaphoretic.	Spasmodic, harsh dry cough, e.g. croup, asthma, pertussis, pleurisy. Hypertension. Hepatitis. Convulsions. Intestinal spasm.	
Marrubium vulgare	Clearing, stimulating, relaxing, cooling. Bitter. Pungent. Salty. Cool.	Stimulating expectorant with amphoteric action. Discharges hyperaemia and congestion. Bitter, stimulant for the liver and gastrointestinal system. Rising hepatic heat affecting the throat.	Acute and chronic bronchitis, sore throats, asthma, especially where there is copious catarrh. Regulates bowel function through bitter action.	Specific for obstructed, deficient, toxic constitutions.
Prunus serotina				Calming and resolvent for heat conditions affecting the lungs.
Primula vera				
Pulmonaria officinalis	Restoring, cleansing.	Mild, restoring tonic for irritable and inflammatory conditions of the lungs. Demulcent.	Acute and chronic cough and inflammatory conditions. Long term restorative.	
Solidago virgaurea	Restoring, astringing, decongesting. Bitter. Astringent. Cool.	Stimulating tonic, astringent and antiseptic for the mucous membranes, particularly for chronic, deficient bronchial conditions.	Bronchitis with purulent catarrhal discharge. Nasopharyngeal catarrh. Hay fever. Acute or chronic kidney disease and infection.	

(Continued)

Herb	Therapeutic movement	Principal therapeutic actions	Conditions applicable and combinations	Energetic actions and notes
		Diuretic, decongestant and restorative for the kidneys.	Oedema from kidney deficiency.	
Thymus vulgaris	Stimulating, restoring. Pungent. Bitter. Astringent.	Stimulating, relaxing, restorative for cold, damp, depleted conditions of the lungs and digestive tract. A secretolytic stimulant expectorant and relaxant. Diaphoretic. Immunological stimulant and restorative. Antiseptic. Adrenal stimulant and restorative.	Acute and chronic lung infections. Bronchitis. Asthma, wheezing, spasmodic cough. Viral, fungal, bacterial infection. Circulatory for cold and damp, rheumatic joints and muscles. Deficient digestion with wind, loose bowels, undigested food, phlegm. General fatigue and immune weakness and specific for lung and digestive weakness.	Refer and contrast with Salvia, Hyssopus, Oreganum, Rosmarinus. Works on higher CNS centres.
Tussilago farfara	Stimulating, restoring, relaxing. Astringent. Bitter. Sweet. Moist.	Stimulating and soothing expectorant and demulcent. Restorative for chronic inflammatory conditions.	Antitussive, relaxant and expectorant for coughs, wheezing, asthma, pertussis. Chronic pulmonary conditions.	
Verbascum thapsus	Restoring, relaxing. Astringent. Sweet. Cool. Moist.	Stimulating, relaxing, demulcent and alterative. Amphoteric actions for removing mucous and easing spasmodic cough. Moistening. Clears congestive blood heat, resolves swelling, dissipates tumours.	Asthma, wheeze and paroxysmal cough. Irritable, inflamed membranes—hay fever Specifically for chronic, deficient lung conditions as a restorative. Swollen glands, tumours, boils, abscesses, eczema, dermatitis. Mouth, eye and ear inflammation.	Verbascum oil—topical.

Respiratory case histories
Case history: sore throat

This 30-year-old man, presents with an acute sore throat and chesty cough. He has vague flu-like symptoms but no temperature. He has had multiple attacks of acute sore throat over the past two years occurring every few weeks and generally has to take a course of antibiotics to clear them.

He describes his energy as moderate. He plays football and considers himself fairly fit. He has occasional headache and dizzy spells. He suffers from moderate hay fever, which has been worse in 2007. He has a tendency to cold peripheral circulation and often gets hot at night. He finds work very stressful through constraints of time pressure and work load.

Previous medical history:
Childhood history of sore throats.

Investigations:
Blood tests negative. Zinc taste test is low.

Clinical signs:
Blood pressure: 130/80.
Tongue: slightly swollen, pale, anterior heat.

A two tier process of treatment; an acute medicine for the first week to combat potential serious bacterial infection, followed by a tonic medicine to work on the underlying disharmony.

Prescriptions:
Acute formula.
Primary functions and actions.
The patient has periodic acute bacterial infections, which require acute treatment both to relieve unpleasant symptoms and to treat the infection. Actions are required that are directly antibacterial to resolve symptoms. This is a potentially serious infection that requires urgent attention, which in the normal course of events would be treated with medically prescribed antibiotics. An improvement in symptomatology is expected to commence within 2–3 hours of the start of treatment.

Herb	Dosage	Actions
Achillea millefolium	15.00	Diffusive action.
Salvia officinalis	10.00	Antimicrobial. Immune enhancing.
Baptisia tinctoria	15.00	Antimicrobial.
Echinacea angustifolia	40.00	Antimicrobial immune response.
Hydrastis canadensis	5.00	Depurative.

(Continued)

Herb	Dosage	Actions
Phytolacca decandra	10.00	Lymphatic agent. Depurative.
Hypericum perforatum	15.00	Restorative.
Dosage: 5 ml of tincture to be given three or four times daily in a little water.	110.00	

Composition and rationale:
The formula is effective against a wide range of possible bacterial and viral infections with a combination of some principal anti-infective herbs, i.e. Salvia, Baptisia, Echinacea. The actions are both directly anti-infective and indirectly stimulating non-specific immune enhancing, with potential topical actions as a result of direct contact on ingestion between the composition and the infected tissues. The Hydrastis and Phytolacca provide lymphatic and depurative support, aiding in the elimination of toxic immunological complexes and further enhancing immune function. The Achillea and Hypericum provide systemic support and direction. The Achillea serves as a general diffuse herb creating a dynamic of externalisation and protection. The Hypericum has a supportive and protective dynamic for the nervous system as a whole and the autonomic profile.

Constitutional formula:
Primary functions and actions:
The formula is designed to address the constitutional pattern that underlies the reoccurrence of the acute infections. The patient has a long history of sore throats from childhood and the presence of current immune complexes are evident by the heat discernible in the exterior part of his tongue. These are indicative of immune dysfunction and the process of internalisation of immune complexes as 'heat'. This has been traditionally termed a 'rising liver heat' issue and often relates to emotional disturbance in childhood affecting the immune regulation and response. There is congestion of the circulation of blood and energy with a higher than optimum blood pressure and poor blood perfusion, as evidenced by the cold peripheral circulation and pale tongue, which may have led to a deficient immune response and vulnerability to bacterial infection. The congestion is probably caused by work stress, pressure and overworking leading to energy depletion and imbalance within the ANS. The medicine is designed to improve energy levels, raise the immune profile, balance the ANS and resolve the pattern of immunological disharmony.

The formula is designed to work over a period of some 2–3 months, gradually increasing energy levels and immune function and also preventing further attacks of infection.

Herb	Dosage	Actions
Achillea millefolium	15.00	Diffusive.
Salvia officinalis	10.00	Anti-infective. Immune enhancing.
Eleutherococcus senticosis	20.00	Tonic, restorative and regulator.

(Continued)

Herb	Dosage	Actions
Astragalus membraneous	15.00	Tonic and immune tonic.
Schizandra chinensis	10.00	Tonic and dispersing.
Hydrastis canadensis	10.00	Depurative and membrane restorative.
Phytolacca decandra	5.00	Depurative and lymphatic agent.
Hypericum perforatum	15.00	Restorative and harmoniser.
Citrus aurantium flores	10.00	Dispersive and aromatic.
Dosage: 5 ml bid aq ac.		

Composition and rationale:
The key components of the formula are the inclusion of several major tonic herbs, Eleutherococcus, Astragalus and Schizandra, which work synergistically to improve the patient's energy foundation. The Eleutherococcus is primarily a tonic to the endocrine systems, pancreas and liver and assists in the normalisation of the autonomic profile through its regulatory actions on the HPA axis. Astragalus is primarily a tonic for the immune system. Schizandra, in this instance, is primarily working as a diffuse agent for the movement of heat.

The Hydrastis and Phytolacca provide lymphatic and depurative support, aiding the elimination of toxic immunological complexes and further enhancing immune function. The Achillea and Hypericum provide systemic support and direction. The Achillea serves as a general diffuse herb, creating a dynamic of externalisation and protection. The Hypericum has a supportive and protective dynamic for the nervous system as a whole and the autonomic profile. The Citrus is used as an aromatic facilitator for the formula as a whole, lifting the emotional tone, resolving negative emotional impressions and reducing the potential for shock from treatment resolution.

Two weeks:
Blood pressure: 135/70.
Tongue pink with reduced heat.

Sore throat NAD. Warm peripheral circulation and no night sweats. Energy improved. Clear head with no dizziness or headache.

Case history: chronic cough

This retired university lecturer, aged 87, presents with a persistent wheezy chest, which he has had for some three months over the winter months. He complains of an intermittent dry and unproductive cough. He has persistent upper respiratory catarrh, particularly in the mornings. He is prone to colds, which frequently lead to chest infections, and he developed pneumonia two years ago.

He complains of feeling fatigued, particularly in the mornings and evenings, and has aches in his muscles and joints. He feels the cold to his core. This man appears sprightly and very youthful for his age. He is of normal weight. He is sociable, outgoing and communicative, although his voice sounds a little weak. He has led a busy and active life and continues to tend his large garden and do his own DIY on his large house. He was widowed the year before and now lives alone.

Clinical signs:
Blood pressure: 105/75.
Pulse: 65.
Pulse pressure: 30.
CVI: 11,700.
Tongue: pale and swollen base, loose white coating.

Analysis:
The patient has a relatively low autonomic sympathetic output, as demonstrated by the low pulse pressure, systolic blood pressure and pulse rate, and as a consequence the lung energy will be deficient. The deficient lung pattern is shown by the wheeziness, unproductive cough and phlegm. As the deficiency pattern will also relate to a low immune profile, the possibility of pathogenic infection should be considered and guarded against.

Herb	Dosage	Actions
Angelica arcangelica radix	10.00	Dispersive circulatory and aromatic.
Eleutherococcus senticosis	15.00	Foundational tonic to support the lung energy and sympathetic activation.
Astragalus membraneous	15.00	Foundational tonic and immune regulator.
Schizandra	10.00	Adjunct for tonic actions.
Inula helenium	10.00	Aromatic sympathetic activator and immune stimulant for the lungs.
Pulmonaria officinalis	15.00	Pulmonary tissue healer.
Althaea officinale radix	15.00	Pulmonary demulcent.
Thymus officinalis	10.00	Anti-infective. Antispasmodic for the lungs.
Cinnamon zeylanicum	5.00	Aromatic agent.
Dosage: 5 ml tid aq ac.	105.00	

Case history: bronchial catarrh

This 14-year-old male has suffered from hay fever type symptoms of variable intensity for several years and the symptoms have become more acute over the past 12 months. He has chronic sinusitis, bronchial catarrh, sore throat and an irritable and unproductive cough.

He describes his energy as low, although he likes sport and is very active. He experiences frequent headaches and has difficulty with concentration. His mood is often low and he frequently feels anxious. He generally feels hot, especially at night. He is of smart appearance and fashionably dressed. He is of normal weight. He is articulate and communicative and appears a little shy and anxious.

Clinical signs:
Blood pressure: 105/78.
Pulse: 76.
Pulse pressure: 27.
Tongue: pale and swollen base, close white coating, intense red papillae.

Analysis:
The patient has a significant autonomic sympathetic deficiency and parasympathetic excess resulting in mucous membrane hyperaemia, irritability and sensitivity. He has endogenous heat and mucus congestion. The syndrome is most likely due to difficulty with his confidence and capacity to deal with his psycho-social environment.

Herb	*Dosage*	*Actions*
Achillea millefolium	15.00	Circulatory dispersive.
Centella asiatica	15.00	CNS and ANS regulator.
Panax ginseng	20.00	Foundational tonic. The development of personal strength and integrity.
Astragalus membraneous	20.00	Foundational and immunological tonic.
Schizandra chinensis	15.00	Adjunct for tonification.
Agrimonia eupatorium	15.00	Liver tonic and restorative for resolution of liver heat syndrome.
Petroselinum crispum	20.00	Parasympathetic drainer. Antispasmodic.
Verbena officinalis	15.00	Nervine tonic restorative.
Rosmarinus officinalis	15.00	Autonomic regulator. Being manifest.
Dosage: 5 ml bid aq ac.	150.00	

The urinary system

Causative factors

Infection	Bacterial
	Viral
	Fungal
Irritation	Poisons and toxins
	Food sensitivities and allergens
	Iatrogenic, e.g. anti-inflammatories
	Immunological residues from systemic infection
Obstruction	Calculi
	Tumour
Inflammation	Endogenous heat which may relate to trauma and abuse
Fatigue factors	Adrenal fatigue may cause irritation and in the long term CKD (chronic kidney disease)

Autonomic balance regulates function with sympathetic activation decreasing kidney function and micturition and parasympathetic increasing function, as part of the SLUD syndrome. Therefore the urinary tract responds to interventions that modify the autonomic nervous system.

Diuretics

May be compulsory diuretics in the orthodox sense, i.e. lead to increased micturition. Oedema is not necessarily the direct consequence of kidney dysfunction and is more likely to be due to circulatory, cardiac or liver disorder. Diuretics may in some cases act through changing circulatory flow and not through altering tubular reabsorption, which is the mechanism of drug diuretics. A diuretic action is ancillary in many medicinal herbs and vegetables.

Diuretics	Taraxacum officinalis herba. Galium aparine. Juniperis communis. Equisetum arvensis. Parietaria officinalis. Filipendula ulmaria. Betula alba. Petroselinum crispus. Hydrangea arborescens. Collinsonia canadenis. Rubia tinctoria. Ononis spinose. Urtica officinalis herba.
Kidney tonics	Arctostaphylos. Apium graveolums. Alchemilla arvensis. Eupatorium purpureum. Juniperis communis. Parietaria officinalis Caution with stimulating diuretics in CKD.
Kidney trophrestoratives	Alchemilla arvensis. Solidago virgauria. Equisetum arvense. Cynara scolymus. Carduus marianus.
Anti-infectives	Barosma betulina. Arctostaphylos uva-ursi. Juniperis communis. Echinacea angustifolia. Baptisia tinctoria. Vaccinium myrtillus. Essential oils excreted through the kidneys, e.g. Thymus.
Demulcents	Althaea officinalis. Zea mays. Agropyron repens.
Anti-lithics (used as infusion)	Hydrangea arborescens. Eupatorium purpureum. Alchemilla arvensis. Collinsonia canadensis. Rubia tinctorum. Parietaria diffusa.
Anti-enuresis See also demulcents and astringents.	Rhus aromatic. Equisetum arvense. Hypericum perfoliatum.
Astringents	Rhus aromatica. Capsella bursa pastoris. Equisetum arvense.
Circulatory Diaphoretics can play an important role both as diffusives to reduce stress on the kidneys but also to improve elimination through the skin.	Achillea millefolium. Eupatorium perfoliatum. Angelica archangelica. Anemone pulsatilla.

Herbs for kidney function

Herb	Therapeutic movement	Principal therapeutic actions	Conditions applicable and combinations	Energetic actions and notes
Agropyron repens	Soothing, relaxing, restorative.	Soothing, demulcent diuretic. Urinary antiseptic. Promotes the excretion of urates, phosphates and gravel.	For all cases of irritation, inflammation, infection or excitability of the urinary tract and prostate. Clears toxic residues. Specific for backache caused by adrenal and kidney dysfunction.	
Aphanes arvensis	Soothing.	Demulcent diuretic and anti-inflammatory.	Specific for mucous membrane irritation and inflammation—urinary calculi, dysuria. Hepatic and renal oedema.	Specific for endogenous heat eliminated through the kidneys.
Apium graveolens	Stimulating, soothing.	Stimulating, relaxing, antispasmodic, restoring diuretic. Antiseptic and anti-inflammatory.	Irritation, inflammation and infection of the genitourinary tract. Specific for rheumatic conditions and associated sciatica and as a tonic nervine for neurasthenia. Regenerative for the kidneys and liver.	
Arctium lappa	See liver herbs.			
Arctostaphylos	Soothing, circulating.	Stimulating, astringent, antiseptic tonic for the pelvic organs.	Irritation and infection and of the kidneys, bladder, urethra, prostate. For deficiency, congestion and prolapse of the pelvic organs.	

(Continued)

Herb	Therapeutic movement	Principal therapeutic actions	Conditions applicable and combinations	Energetic actions and notes
Barosma betulina	Diffusing.	Stimulating, soothing, diffusive, antiseptic tonic for the pelvic organs. Depurative diuretic.	Oedema. Irritation, inflammation, infection of the renal system, especially associated with chronic atonic and congestive conditions. Pelvic congestion and prolapse.	
Capsella bursa pastoris		Gentle stimulant, relaxant and astringent for the urinary system.	Irritation and congestion of the kidneys. Haemorrhage—haematuria, menorrhagia, metorrhagia, heamoptesis, epistaxis.	
Cynara scolymus	See liver herbs.			
Equisetum arvense	Regulating. Diffusive.	Stimulant, tonic and diuretic to the bladder and kidneys. Improves connective tissue tone. Anti-inflammatory.	Cystitis, urethritis. Torpid and congestive conditions of the pelvic organs including prostate, uterus, bladder. Metabolic oedema. Dispersal of inorganic compounds.	Removal of deep patterns of toxaemia and tissue regeneration.
Eupatorium purpureum	Relaxing. Diffusive.	Gently stimulating and relaxing depurative diuretic. Emmenagogue.	Deficiency, congestion and constriction of the pelvic organs, particularly the kidneys. Chronic cystitis.	

(Continued)

Herb	Therapeutic movement	Principal therapeutic actions	Conditions applicable and combinations	Energetic actions and notes
Galium aparine	Soothing, relaxing.	Relaxing, soothing diuretic.	Irritation, congestion and inflammation of the kidneys and bladder. To assist the removal of toxicity and heat through the kidneys—eczema, psoriasis.	
Juniperis communis	Diffusive. Transformative.	Stimulating, relaxing and antiseptic diuretic.	Kidney congestion and oedema. Stimulating depurative for toxic heat conditions. Contraindicated in parachymal kidney disease and pregnancy.	Transformative agent for toxic heat conditions eliminated through the kidneys.
Rhus aromatica		Stimulating, astringent, tonic for GIT and GUT. Decreases overexcitability.	Polyuria, enuresis, nocturia to reduce overactivity and excitability.	
Solidago virgaurea	Resolvant.	Stimulating, astringent, antiseptic tonic for the mucous membranes. Stimulates renal excretion.	Restorative for acute and chronic kidney disease and associated albuminuria and haematuria.	Resolves and restores tissues affected by deep patterns of disharmony.
Taraxacum officinalis herba	Transformative. Restorative.	Stimulating and soothing diuretic.	Oedema. Specific for the removal of uric acid and in the treatment of arthritic and rheumatic conditions.	

(Continued)

Herb	Therapeutic movement	Principal therapeutic actions	Conditions applicable and combinations	Energetic actions and notes
Urtica dioica	Restorative, soothing.	Anti-inflammatory, antiseptic, antiallergic, depurative diuretic. Blood tonic and restorative.	Oedema. Cystitis. Depurative diuretic for toxic heat conditions—eczema, acne, urticaria, furunculosis and uric acid. Specific for prostatic hypertrophy and carcinoma.	
Zea mays	Soothing.	Demulcent for the kidneys and bladder.	For irritation and inflammation of the kidneys and bladder. Enuresis.	

Case history: irritable bladder

A 38-year-old female teaching assistant presents with dysuria and frequency, which she has had for some 18 months. She has chronic lower abdominal soreness, which is worse with micturition, and also has intermittent episodes of very acute symptoms, sometimes with blood and mucous. She reports feeling very anxious and has low energy. She has a previous history of IBS and has suffered recurrent attacks of vaginal thrush. Her menstrual cycle is a regular 28 days and of normal flow and duration.

Clinical signs:
Blood pressure: 120/80.
Pulse: 84.
Pulse pressure: 40.

Analysis:
The patient suffers from an irritable bladder, but has attacks of bacterial cystitis from time to time, which she has treated with antibiotics. She has a slight sympathetic deficiency and excess parasympathetic condition with some smooth muscle constraint. The syndrome is most likely compounded by fatigue factors. The herbal intervention is designed to regulate the autonomic nervous system and provide foundational support and resources.

Herb	Dosage	Actions
Angelica archangelica radix	10.00	Aromatic circulatory.
Centella asiatica	20.00	CNS and ANS balancer. Adaptogen.
Codonopsis pilosa	30.00	Foundational tonic and adaptogen.

(Continued)

Herb	Dosage	Actions
Lycium barabarum	15.00	Liver tissue tonic and restorative.
Iris versicolor	15.00	Liver stimulant for liver heat. The cultivation of female inspiration and creativity.
Rosa damascena	15.00	Liver heat remedy. Transformation of liver heat.
Stachys betonica	20.00	Cerebral-spinal restorative.
Verbena officinalis	15.00	Nerve restorative.
Salvia triloba	10.00	Autonomic regulator. Manifestation of self.
	150.00	

Remedy for acute bacterial cystitis

Herb	Dosage	Actions
Achillea millefolium	15.00	Diffusive circulatory agent.
Barosma betulina	30.00	Stimulating diuretic. Anti-infective agent.
Arctostaphylos uva-ursi	20.00	Diuretic. Anti-infective. Astringent.
Alchemilla arvensis	20.00	Soothing diuretic and demulcent.
Zea mays	20.00	Demulcent.
Dosage: 5 ml qid aq when required.	155.00	

Case history: kidney stones

A 68-year-old male wood joiner complains of persistent soreness in the left lower quadrant of his abdomen for the past few weeks. He has frequency of micturition, nocturia and his urine has a dark and concentrated appearance. He is generally fatigued but otherwise in good general health.

Clinical signs:
Blood pressure: 150/90.
Pulse: 68.
Pulse pressure: 60.

Analysis:
The patient is most likely to be dehydrated, judging by the appearance of his urine, and this is most likely to be a key causative factor. He also has relatively high diastolic blood pressure, which denotes a generalised spastic status of his smooth muscle, which would include the kidney ducts and result in impediment to urinary flow.

The intervention is to move the circulation and relax the smooth muscle, stimulate the urinary tract to improve urinary flow, and promote anti-inflammatory and anti-infective actions.

Herb	Dosage	Actions
Achillea millefolium	15.00	Circulatory diffusive.
Eucommia ulmoides	20.00	Foundation tonic. Hypotensive.
Schizandra chinensis	10.00	Adjunct for tonification.
Barosma betulina	15.00	Stimulating and relaxing diuretic.
Agropyron repens	15.00	Anti-inflammatory. Kidney restorative.
Urtica officinalis radix	15.00	Anti-inflammatory. Relaxing diuretic.
Zea mays	15.00	Urinary tract demulcent.
Dosage: 5 ml tid.	105.00	

Following the remedy, the patient passed pieces of gravel after two weeks, which resolved the problem.

The female reproductive system

Irritation

The same principals of reflex action and irritation apply as with other systems, e.g. leucorrhoea may be a non-infected, irritable and spasmodic condition related to parasympathetic over-activity.

Hormone levels

Oestrogen promotes emotion and testosterone promotes activation and libido.

Oestrogen dominance

Oestrogen dominance occurs when the body is producing too much oestrogen in relation to progesterone. Progesterone is only produced following ovulation and ovulation doesn't occur with the oral contraceptive pill or following menopause. Levels of progesterone in these situations are very low compared with oestrogen levels. Oestrogen is also produced by fat cells, the adrenal glands and the brain:

> Breast tenderness, endometriosis, uterine fibroids, increased risk of breast and uterine cancers.
> Fibrocystic breasts, mood swings and depression, irritability, nervousness and anxiety, poor concentration, migraine, weight gain, water retention, fatigue, sugar cravings, severe pre-menstrual syndrome, heavy and irregular periods.

Insufficient oestrogen

The opposite situation can also occur, where there is insufficient oestrogen compared with progesterone. Typical symptoms of oestrogen deficiency include:

> Hot flushes, night sweats, poor memory, tearfulness and depression, mood swings, vaginal dryness, painful intercourse, low libido, palpitations, urinary incontinence, bone loss, dry skin, headache, sleep disturbances.

DHEA (dehydroepiandrosterone)

A precursor for testosterone and oestrogen. DHEA is affected by stress, by increased cortisol levels and decreased serotonin. A decrease in DHEA will also result in impaired immune function.

Testosterone

Testosterone is an important hormone for males and females, although in less quantity in females. It is important for activation and energy. Deficiency causes the following:

> Decreased motivation, anxiety and depression, fatigue, lack of focus, decreased sense of well-being, muscular aches and pains, bone loss, allergies, decreased sweating.

Hormone levels are affected by stress, diet, and other exogenous factors. For example, exposure to xenoestrogens from plastics, heavy metals in the body, exposure to pesticides, food additives, such as aspartame and MSG, excess oestrogen from dairy, growth hormones from meat.

Oestrogen is effective in most tissues in the body and is a significant factor in reducing inflammation in many diseases (Vageto et al., 2002).

Constitutional dynamics

Hormone regulation	Control of the hormone cycle is via hypothalamic/pituitary regulation. The HPA axis in response to stress decreases sex hormone secretion. Sex hormones promote serotonin secretion and vice versa. The HPT axis is affected by hormone deficiency, both sex and adrenal: depletion syndromes generally involve a combination of deficiency of sex hormones, thyroid, adrenal cortical and associated with passive sympathetic deficiency.

(Continued)

Blood dynamics	Normal menstruation requires sufficient blood and free circulation. Free circulation is dependent upon the ANS and the effects of liver function.
Pelvic congestion and pain result from blood stagnation, in particular from constraint associated with emotional tension.
Pelvic congestion also arises from blood stagnation from deficiency or weakness, e.g. from central depletion or deficiency within the endocrine system and also from issues with blood quality and volume.
The circulatory dynamics are significantly affected by the menstrual cycle, e.g. there is usually a significant blood deficiency pre-menstrually.
Hormone deficiency significantly affects the blood dynamics with vasoconstriction causing elevation of the diastolic blood pressure.
Autonomic balance	ANS balance and regulation. The effects of sympathetic tone on vasoconstriction. Sympathetic passive deficiency and depletion leads to pelvic pooling of blood and visceroptosis.
Heat conditions	Liver heat syndrome is often implicated in inflammatory issues and infection in the reproductive system, e.g. PID—inflammation, infection and pelvic pooling of blood.
Pre-menstrual tension	Pre-menstrual tension may relate to underlying emotional tension, blood deficiency or sympathetic deficiency and may be an exacerbation of underlying tension. Normally the frontal cortex regulates vascular tension prevent or reducing pre-menstrual tension.

Relationship to other organ systems

- There is an intimate relationship of nervous innervation with the lower back. Chronic lower back problems frequently follow the menopause.
- There is a strong association with the urinary system, with disturbance in one often referring to the other, with the same herbs applying to both systems.
- Similarly the digestive tract.
- The protein sex hormone binding globulin is produced by the liver and binds hormones to limit quantities in the blood.
- High insulin levels are related to excess oestrogen secretion and high oestrogen levels are associated with weight increase. Metabolic syndrome and insulin resistance in PCOS.
- Adrenal stimulation causes increased testosterone secretion in line with other hormones—cortisol, glucocorticoids, DHEA and the synthesis of adrenal sex hormones. Testosterone is associated with activation, oestrogen with emotion.
- Liver function determines the availability of materials for hormone synthesis, e.g. B vitamins, essential fatty acids.

Herbal actions for the female reproductive system

Relaxants Applicable to spasmodic conditions of the uterus and associated structures. Tension may be physiologically induced, e.g. from hormone deficiency or psychogenic. Physiological conditions respond to physiological interventions but psychogenic conditions respond best to interventions at the limbic level. Dysmenorrhoea may be spastic or congestive. Spastic is related primarily to smooth muscle contractibility, congestive relates to pelvic and uterine congestion.	Anemone pulsatilla, Angelica archangelica, Caulophyllum, Dioscorea villosa, Mitchella, Viburnum opulus, Cimicifuga racemosa, Leonorus cardiacca, Chamomilla, Viscum alba.
Hormone regulators ANS and hypothalamic balancers. Pituitary regulators.	Panax ginseng, Codonopsis, Salvia triloba, Rosmarinus officinalis, Smilax ornate, Centella asiatica. Chamaelerium luteum, Vitex agnus castus, Dioscorea villosa, Alchemilla vulgaris. Chamaelerium and Dioscorea are regarded as oestrogenic, Vitex as progesteronenic.
Reproductive tonics Stimulating and relaxing to the uterus and ovaries and tonic to the pelvic tissues. Improve cerebral-spinal tone.	Aletris, Chamaelerium, Mitchella, Caulophyllum, Trigonella, Serenoa, Angelica sinensis, Cimicifuga, Rubus, Viburnum prunifolium, Calendula
Emmenagogues Stimulating and tonic to the uterus.	Artemisia spp., Ruta, Achillea, Salvia officinalis, Juniperis officinalis, Rosmarinus officinalis, Mentha spp.
Astringents Applicable to menorrhagia and to improve tone and ascend function. Menorrhagia may be due to congestion, obstruction, infection or disorders of the circulatory system (anaemia, capillary fragility, coagulation defects etc.) Astringents in the Rose family are particularly helpful for resolution of emotionally charged conditions.	Achillea Trillium, Geranium, Hydrastis, Nymphae, Myrica, Capsella bursa pastoris, Mitchella Rubus.
Ascending herbs For visceroptosis and organ prolapse.	Tonics Astringents, e.g. .Agrimonia, Geranium. Stimulant/astringents, e.g. Myrica, Cimicifuga racemose.

Herbs for the reproductive system

Herb	Therapeutic movement	Principal therapeutic actions	Conditions applicable and combinations	Energetic actions and notes
Alchemilla vulgaris	Relaxing, decongesting, restoring. Bitter, astringent.	Astringent tonic for the uterus and respiratory membranes. Haemostatic. Depurative. Emmenagogue.	Menorrhagia, metrorrhagia, fibroids. **Special features: progesteronal tonic and astringent for the female reproductive system.** Tonic for breast tissue. Astringent for vaginal discharge, leucorrhoea. Astringent tonic for the respiratory membranes.	Toxic blood heat factors affecting the uterus.
Aletris farinosa	Restoring, harmonising. Bitter, astringent.	Uterine tonic. Bitter, stomachic. Cerebral-spinal restorative.	Amenorrhoea, dysmenorrhoea, menstrual irregularity. Nervous dyspepsia, anorexia. Stimulating tonic for the female reproductive system to improve sexual function, sterility and tissue tone especially related to the menopause. Improves circulatory deficiency and cerebral circulation subsequent to hormone dysfunction. Prevents miscarriage.	Promotion of the feminine essence, grace and beauty. Intimacy through sexuality.
Angelica sinensis	Restoring, stimulating and relaxing. Warm, dry, bitter, pungent, sweet.	Circulatory tonic. Diaphoretic. Antispasmodic, carminative. Antibacterial, antifungal, antiseptic. Bitter, diuretic, cholagogue.	Circulatory insufficiency Vascular disease—intermittent claudication. Headache and migraine, respiratory infections, brochitis, coughs, asthma. Dyspepsia, appetite stimulant, alcoholism.	Differentiate from Angelica archangelica. Available in prepared form, i.e. honey baked.

(Continued)

Herb	Therapeutic movement	Principal therapeutic actions	Conditions applicable and combinations	Energetic actions and notes
			Menopausal symptoms, specifically: Tonic for nervous exhaustion, neurasthenia and associated problems with headache, deficient peripheral and cerebral circulation, liver congestion. Specific action to build the quality of the blood. Is said to harmonise the blood. Regulates blood sugar. Hormone balancing and uterine tonification. Specific for amenorrhoea, dysmenorrhoea, metrorrhagia, PMS, menopausal symptoms, infertility and problems with libido. Action of the uterus is amphoteric—relieves spasm of dilation. Immunological stimulant— increases phagocytosis and lymphocytosis.	
Artemisia vulgaris	Stimulating, decongesting, restoring. Bitter, pungent.	Uterine stimulant and restorative. Antiseptic, anti-inflammatory.	Stimulates uterine tone and blood, specific for amenorrhoea associated with blood stagnation.	
Calendula officinalis	Decongesting, softening, astringing. Bitter, sweet, salty, pungent.	Vulnerary, cleansing, anti-inflammatory action. Decongestant and deobstruent. Lymphatic agent. Anticancer.	Tissue healing and repair and the treatment of a wide range of inflammatory and infectious conditions. Resolvent, cleansing, stimulating action specific for liver congestion with associated pelvic and portal congestion.	

(Continued)

Herb	Therapeutic movement	Principal therapeutic actions	Conditions applicable and combinations	Energetic actions and notes
			linked with headache, venous stasis, fibroids and tumours. Oestrogenic.	
Caulophylum thalictroides	Stimulating, relaxing, restoring, decongesting. Bitter, pungent, sweet.	Antispasmodic. Uterine tonic. Nervine. Anti-inflammatory. Diaphoretic. Diuretic.	Antispasmodic for ovaritis, dysmenorrhoea, urethritis, vaginitis as well as migraine, hypertension, palpitation, intestinal cramps. Amenorrhoea. Stimulating, relaxing and diffusive tonic for the uterus and all spastic conditions. Improves circulatory balance and deficient cerebral flow subject to hormonal dysfunctional. Specific for reproductive and circulatory spasm and irritability as a result of the menopause. Co-ordinates uterine contractions during pregnancy and child birth—stimulates contractions where deficient in child birth, relaxes over contraction in false labour pains.	
Chamaelerium lutea	Restoring, stabilising, cutting. Bitter, astringent.	Reproductive tonic. CNS trophorestorative. Diuretic, hepatic.	Amenorrhoea, dysmenorrhoea, menorrhagia. Partus preparator, threatened miscarriage. Stimulating tonic for deficient function of the female and male reproductive systems.	

(Continued)

Herb	Therapeutic movement	Principal therapeutic actions	Conditions applicable and combinations	Energetic actions and notes
Mitchella repens	Restoring, astringing, decongesting. Astringent, bitter, cool.	Uterine tonic. Astringent. Alterative. Diuretic.	Partus preparator. Post-partum haemorrhage. Dysmenorrhoea. Dysuria, oedema. Stimulating tonic for debility of the pelvic organs particularly the uterus; uterine prolapse, menorrhagia.	
Rubus idaeus	Astringing, restoring. Astringent, cool, dry.	Gentle acting, soothing astringent tonic.	Partus preparatus. Menorrhagia. Irritated membranes— leucorrhoea, acute and chronic diarrhoea, summer diarrhoea, laryngitis, pharyngitis.	
Serenoa repens	Restoring. Pungent, sweet, astringent.	Endocrine tonic Genitourinary tonic and alterative. Diuretic, urinary antiseptic. Endocrine stimulant. Antispasmodic, sedative. Expectorant, anti-inflammatory. Depurative.	Male and female sterility, impotence and sexual dysfunction. Gentio-urinary tract infection—PID, ovaritis, salpingitis, orchitis, epididymitis, prostatitis, cystitis. Prostatic hypertrophy, carcinoma. Uterine enlargement. Underdeveloped breast development. Polycystic ovary disease (PCOS). **Special features: a stimulating depurative tonic for the male and female reproductive and urinary systems for deficiency, congestion and infection. For infertility and deficient sexual activity and development in both sexes.**	

(Continued)

Herb	Therapeutic movement	Principal therapeutic actions	Conditions applicable and combinations	Energetic actions and notes
			Serenoa prevents the production of dihydro-testosterone (DHT) from testosterone.	
Trillium pendulum	Stimulating, relaxing, restoring, cutting. Pungent, sour, sweet, astringent.	Genitourinary tonic. Astringent, antihemorrhagic. Antiseptic, antifungal. Alterative.	Menorrhagia, metrorrhagia, vaginal discharge, leucorrhoea. Haematuria. Diarrhoea, dysentery, pectoral. Astringent tonic for mucous membrane inflammation and irritation and to strengthen the pelvic organs; specifically for menopausal menorrhagia, uterine haemorrhage and prolapse. Promotes central strength and relieves congestion.	
Turnera diffusa	Stimulating, restoring. Bitter, pungent.	CNS stimulant. Aphrodisiac. Nerve trophorestorative, thymoleptic. Diuretic. Laxative.	Stimulant to the digestive tract—dyspepsia, constipation. Enuresis, irritable bladder. Prostatic hypertrophy. Amenorrhoea, dysmenorrhoea. Premature ejaculation and sexual weakness. **Special features: stimulating tonic, restorative and balancer for the CNS and ANS in depressed, debilitated and deficient conditions and with particular connection to the generative system. Impotence, sexual deficiency and sexual dysfunction in both sexes.**	

(Continued)

Herb	Therapeutic movement	Principal therapeutic actions	Conditions applicable and combinations	Energetic actions and notes
Viburnum prunifolium	Relaxing, restoring, stabilising. Bitter, astringent, dry.	Antispasmodic. Astringent. Diuretic. Sedative, analgesic.	Stimulating, astringent and relaxing tonic for the genitourinary systems—uterine prolapse, menopausal weakness and menorrhagia. Morning sickness, partus preparator, post-partum haemorrhage, false labour pains. Antispasmodic for all conditions of colic and spasm—hypertension, cramp, asthma. Dysmenorrhoea, menorrhagia, metrorrhagia. Diarrhoea. Anxiety, panic.	
Vitex agnus castus		Hormone adaptogen.	Amenorrhoea, dysmenorrhoea, infertility, PMS Mastitis, mastalgia. Prostatic hypertrophy. Has an amphoteric action upon the pituitary to regulate function—applicable to imbalance of production of releasing hormones, sexual (increases LH, decreases FH), TSH, prolactin. Hyperprolactinaemia, PCOS, endometriosis, fluid retention, breast swelling with PMS. Conditions of hypo-oestrogen, hyper-oestrogen, hypo-progesterone.	

Case history: uterine fibroids

This patient, aged 31, presented with uterine fibroids. Her menstrual cycle is irregular, generally of 15 to 16 days but previously was a regular 28 days. She has menorrhagia with an eight day flow with the first two days very heavy. She has a fibroid which has been assessed as some 6 to 7 cm.

General constitution:
Head 'foggy', has frequent headaches and some unsteadiness. She feels distant and disconnected. She has a stiff neck and shoulders. She has cold peripheral circulation and feels very cold to the core. She often feels 'shaky'. Her digestion is turbulent and bloated and she is inclined to constipation. Wheat, wine and coffee aggravate her digestive symptoms. Blood tests reveal iron deficiency anaemia for which she takes Floradix.

Clinical signs:
Blood pressure: 110/76.
Pulse: 96. Pulse pressure: 34.
CVI: 17,856.

General:
This woman is well-groomed, fashionably dressed, attractive and of slim build. She is wearing many layers of clothing. Her hands are cold despite being in a warm room. Her skin is clear. It is difficult to ascertain skin perfusion, due to her skin colour. She is sociable and articulate. She is of Portuguese origin but speaks fluent English. She was accompanied by her husband who is also of Portuguese origin and seems very supportive. She is confident and assertive but seems tense. Her eyes are 'glassy'.

Herb	Dosage	Actions
Achillea millefolium	15.00	Uterine astringent and tissue restorative. Eases uterine and pelvic blood congestion. Free and easy movement.
Centella asiatica	15.00	Structure, regulation and foundation through regulation of the ANS, CNS and hypothalamus.
Codonopsis pilosula	20.00	Foundation energy through tonification of the endocrine system. Regulation of blood sugar. Promotion of blood production. Promotion of assertion and authority.
Lycium barbarum	10.00	Sweet, nourishing foundation and tissue tonic for the liver and endocrine system. Promotes the resolution of heat. Eases false fire and promotes the constructive expression of 'fire'.

(Continued)

Herb	Dosage	Actions
Iris versicolor	10.00	Hepatic, lymphatic and alterative for endogenous heat and congestion. Promotion of the feminine creative, intuitive process and the relationship to the etheric portal.
Paeonia laterifolia	15.00	Cooling for endogenous heat. Liver tissue rejuvenation. 'Blooming' of the inner beauty.
Glycyrrhiza glabra	15.00	Nourishing foundation tonic for the adrenals, liver and pancreas.
Vitex agnus castus	15.00	Pituitary regulation of the hormonal systems.
Aletrisa farinosa	10.00	Promotion of the feminine essence, grace and beauty. Intimacy through sexuality.
Rubus idaeus	15.00	Uterine tonic, astringent and restorative. The Rose principle applied to endogenous heat invading the reproductive system.
Rosmarinus officinalis	15.00	Autonomic regulation. Regulation of the digestive system. On being manifest. In the world but not of the world.
Dosage: 5 ml bid aq ac.	150.00	

Follow up information

Week	BP	Pulse	Pulse pressure	Symptoms	Tongue
0	110/76	96	34		Very pale.
2	116/70	88	46		
6	106/62		44	MC regular. Heavy menstruation.	
8	110/70		40	MC 28 days, menstruation less heavy.	
12	110/66	74	44	MC 27 days. Seven-day flow, less heavy.	Pink anterior.

Following this the patient was very emotional for two weeks and had been reviewing her abusive childhood experiences and relationship with her father and step-mother. Her father told her when she was 14 that he didn't love her and never had done. She cannot understand why she continues to visit them and be polite when she goes to see family in Portugal. She didn't wish to continue with the tincture but would like help with her emotions. A formulation of Bach flower essences was prepared.

Bach flower essence in rose tincture

Agrimony	Acceptance and peace in the presence of life's trials and difficulties.
Holly	Helps gain perspective of internal negative emotions and conflicts. Love and gentleness.
Walnut	Freedom, self-determination. Protection from outside influences
Cherry Plum	Mental strain and fear of losing one's reason. Letting go and letting God.
Wild Rose	For resignation. Brings back the joy and spirit of life.

7 drops four times daily

One month:
The patient felt much benefit emotionally and felt that she had come to terms with her childhood experience. She was contemplating visiting her father to ask him why he behaved as he did to her.

Case history: endometriosis, anxiety

The patient, aged 42, complains of persistent low level anxiety, which is not provoked by any particular situation. She has experienced the problem for most of her life but it has become worse over the last two years. She has a happy family life and her social and work circumstances are not problematical. The patient is concerned with moderately severe acne on her face. This can sometimes by cystic and painful. She has had the condition since her teens.

General constitution:
The patient describes her energy as generally good. She feels warm both in her body and to her peripheries. She rarely has a headache but reports some problems with memory and focus. Her neck and shoulders are described as tight, especially when she has PMT. The patient is well-groomed and fashionably dressed. She is of normal weight. She is articulate and sociable and perhaps a little shy.

MC: Regular cycle and normal flow. Some PMT and mood swings related to her hormones. A recent gynaecological check-up together with a scan revealed no abnormalities (including the endometriosis referred to in the notes below).

Clinical signs:
Blood pressure: 100/62.
Pulse: 70.
Pulse pressure: 38.

This woman had been treated with herbal medicine 13 years previously, over a period of 3–4 years for endometriosis. This had been identified by laparoscopy as bilateral and associated with the ovaries. She had menorrhagia and dysmenorrhoea with a flow of 5–7 days. She had significant PMT for 7–10 days. She had regular spotting. She has two children of 4 and 6. She ceased the contraceptive pill six years previously.

Blood pressure: 105/70.
Pulse 68.
Pulse pressure: 35.
Tongue: swollen, colour moderate, anterior heat papillae, dry.

Previous medication for endometriosis:
Angelica sinensis 15
Centella 15
Lycium 10
Iris 10
Paeonia 12.5
Carbenia 15
Vitex 15
Chamaelerium 12.5
Calendula 15
Pelagonium 5
Achillea 15

Current medication:
Angelica sinensis 20
Centella 15
Condonopsis 30
Lycium 15
Iris 15
Paeonia 15
Glycyrrhiza 20
Aletris 10
Rosa 10

Case history: dysmenorrhoea, menorrhagia

This woman, aged 26, presented with a history of dysmenorrhoea and menorrhagia. For some 6–7 years her menstrual cycle has tended to be late and heavy and painful with clotting. The flow lasts for 5–6 days. She has a dull, muzzy head for most of the time with frequent acute headaches. She nearly always has an acute headache or migraine at the onset of menstruation. Migraines are accompanied by hot flashes and numbness in her hands.

Her digestion has been problematic for the past four years with intermittent episodes of sickness and diarrhoea. She also experiences general bloating and discomfort often. She is of the opinion that wheat and milk products don't agree with her.

She reports her energy as being poor. She has cold peripheral circulation to the hands and feet but often feels hot at night. She has moderate acne on her face which is worse during menstruation.

Clinical signs:
Blood pressure: 134/82.
Pulse: 76.
Pulse pressure: 52.
Tongue: slight pale base, close white coating. Red papillae in the tip.

This woman communicates easily and articulates herself well but appears slightly shy. She is appreciably over weight and has noticeably pronounced hair on her arms. She is unmarried and works in the office of the family business.

Herb	Dosage	Actions
Angelica sinensis	15.00	Blood and hormone tonic.
Centella asiatica	15.00	CNS and ANS balancer.
Schizandra	10.00	Adjunct for tonic actions. Regulation of 'fire'.
Chicorium intybus	15.00	Dispersive for liver heat and false fire.
Paeonia lactiflora alba	15.00	Regulator for liver heat and function.
Matricaria recutita	15.00	Visceral smooth muscle relaxant.
Polygonum multiflorum	20.00	Foundational tonic.
Rosa damascena	10.00	Resolution of heat and emotional tension.
Plantago lanceolata	15.00	Demulcent for resolution of endogenous heat.
Verbena officinalis	10.00	Nervine restorative.
Citrus aurantium flores	10.00	Aromatic facilitator.
Dosage: 5 ml bid.	150.00	

Case history: infertility

This lady of 36-years-old has had four miscarriages all at around six weeks of pregnancy. Her general energy is described as reasonable. She has frequent headache. Menstrual cycle is 28 days in a regular cycle. She has moderate to severe PMS for one week.

Clinical signs:
Blood pressure: 110/80.
Pulse: 72.
Pulse pressure: 30.
Tongue: very pale and swollen with anterior heat.

This patient has two syndromes, which are inter-related; a significant deficiency condition and an endogenous heat syndrome, both of which may be problematical to pregnancy. The choice of herbs in the formulation needs careful consideration as the patient may become pregnant whilst taking the medicine.

Herb	Dosage	Actions
Angelica sinensis	20.00	Blood and hormone tonic.
Centella asiatica	15.00	CNS/ANS regulator. Anti-inflammatory.
Codonopsis pilosa	30.00	Foundation tonic.
Schizandra chinensis	10.00	Adjunct to support tonic and anti-inflammatory herbs.
Aletris farinosa	10.00	Regulator for ovarian function.
Glycyrrhiza glabra	15.00	Hormonal foundational tonic.
Vitex agnus castus	15.00	Pituitary hormone regulator.
Rehmannia glutinosa prep.	25.00	Foundation hormone tonic.
Citrus aurantium flores	10.00	Aromatic facilitator.
Dosage: 5 ml bid.	150.00	

The patient took the medicine for three months at which point she became pregnant. She ultimately had a healthy pregnancy and gave birth to a baby boy.

Case history: hot flushes

This lady aged 51, has experienced severe hot flushes night and day for five months. She has a hysterectomy 14 years ago, but not oophorectomy, for menorrhagia. No HRT taken. She has a history of breast lumps. Very fatigued. She was diagnosed as suffering from type 2 diabetes two years ago and this is controlled with diet. She was diagnosed with asthma six years previously. She has cold peripheral circulation.

Clinical signs:
Blood pressure: 140/85.
Tongue: pale, swollen, slippery with anterior heat.

Triad formulation for hot flushes:
Salvia triloba—10 (pituitary regulation for follicle stimulating hormone (FSH) regulation)
Aletris—10 (ovarian regulation)
Cimicifuga—10 (cerebral-spinal restorative)

Dosage: 30 ml. 15 drops bid.

Case history: pre-menstrual tension

This lady, aged 38, has been suffering from pre-menstrual tension for over ten years. Symptoms last for some ten days, with bloating, breast tenderness and fluid retention, severe emotional upset and feeling of being clumsy, headachy and agitated. She also has lower backache. Her menstrual cycle is a regular 28 days with a flow of about 5 days, which is heavy to start with. She has some dysmenorrhoea. She has been diagnosed as having a small fibroid.

She reports her energy as being low and says she feels very 'stressed'. She experiences frequent sinus type of headache. Her digestion is reported as normal with normal bowel movements. She has an intermittent sore throat. She describes herself as hot, particularly at night.

Clinical signs:
Blood pressure: 110/80.
Pulse: 98.
Pulse pressure: 30.
Tongue: normal pink colouration, slight dry and anterior heat papillae.

Medication:
Self-administered—Vitex agnus castus, B6, evening primrose oil.

This patient has a significantly low pulse pressure but note should be taken of the stage of her hormone cycle when her blood pressure was taken, as pre-menstrually she has a blood deficiency condition. Pre-menstrual tension is normally associated with a progesterone deficiency, which in turn is related to an autonomic deficiency. She has a slight oestrogen dominance due to the progesterone deficiency. She also has a degree of vasoconstriction. Dependent upon where she is in her menstrual cycle, this may be related to the pre-menstrual tension or it may be contributory to it. The medicine is formulated to provide endocrine augmentation and regulation and autonomic balance.

Herb	Dosage	Actions
Angelica sinensis	20.00	Promotion of blood movement. Hormone and blood tonic.
Centella asiatica	15.00	CNS and ANS regulator.
Schizandra chinensis	10.00	Adjunct for tonics. Regulation of 'fire'.
Turnera	15.00	Anabolic tonic.
Taraxacum officinalis radix	20.00	Foundational tonic and adaptogen.
Paeonia laterifolia alba	15.00	Liver heat regulator.
Carbenia benedictus	15.00	Liver restorative and regulator. Cerebral-spinal restorative.
Verbena officinalis	15.00	Nervine.
Hyssopus officinalis	15.00	Nervine. Autonomic relaxant and regulator.
Citrus flores	10.00	Aromatic facilitator.
Dosage: 5 ml bid.	150.00	

Case history: menopausal hot flushes

This menopausal lady has been suffering from severe and frequent hot flushes, which are worse at night, since stopping HRT three months previously. She was unhappy with HRT because of break through bleeding, gaining weight and abdominal bloating. She also suffers from memory loss, poor concentration and some depression. She has had amenorrhoea for 18 months. She reports her energy as reasonable. She also has some mild asthma and hay fever.

Clinical signs:
Blood pressure: L: 145/95. R: 145/93.
Pulse: 86.
Tongue: swollen with moderate colour and anterior red papillae.

Herb	Dosage	Actions
Anemone pulsatilla	15.00	Circulatory regulator. Antispasmodic for hormone deficiency.
Salvia triloba	10.00	CNS and ANS balancer. Pituitary hormone regulator.
Schizandra chinensis	15.00	Adjunct for tonic actions.
Lycium barbarum	15.00	Adjunct for tonic actions. Liver foundational tonic.
Artemisia vulgaris	10.00	Transformation agent for endogenous heat.
Leonorus	15.00	Antispasmodic for hormone deficiency symptoms.
Alchemilla vulgaris	15.00	Hormonal facilitator.
Rehmannia glutinosa prep.	20.00	Foundational nutritional tonic.
Polygonum multiflorum	15.00	Foundational endocrine tonic.
Chamaelerium, lutea	10.00	Ovarian regulator. Cerebral-spinal restorative.
Pelargonium graveolums	10.00	Aromatic facilitator.
Dosage: 5 ml bid.	150.00	

The male reproductive system

Libido

Libido is directly related to energy status, circulatory dynamics and ANS balance; the maintenance of a vital sympathetic tone in the autonomic nervous system is essential. Men typically experience problems with libido following life changing events, which affect the autonomic nervous system, e.g. retirement.

Prostate hyperplasia

Prostatic hypertrophy—non-infective enlargement through hormonal change, differentiated from irritable bladder, prostatitis and prostate cancer.

Benign prostatic hypertrophy (BPH) is a complex condition, which is not fully understood but has definite links with changes in hormonal levels, inflammation and stress and fatigue factors.

Androgens are necessary for BPH to occur but do not directly cause the condition. Castrated boys do not develop BPH in the way that intact men do, and administration of androgens does not worsen the condition. There is evidence that a metabolite of testosterone, dihydro-testosterone (DHT), produced by the enzyme 5α-reductase, type 2, is a major factor in hyperplasia. DHT is ten times more potent than testosterone because is dissociates from androgen receptors more slowly. This is evidenced by the fact that an inhibitor of enzyme 5α-reductase is effective in the treatment of BHP (Sun et al., 2011). Serenoa is the herb of choice for reducing the production of DHT.

There is evidence that oestrogens are involved in the aetiology of BPH. Men with BPH generally have elevated levels of oestrogens and reduced free testosterone levels. Cells from the prostates of men with BPH grow in response to high oestradiol levels and low testosterone.

It is possible that oestrogens render cells more susceptible to the actions of DHT. It is likely that it is not the presence of higher levels of oestrogen as such that causes the problem but rather the ratio of oestrogen to testosterone (Braun & Anderson, 2011). Low testosterone is associated with low endocrine function and fatigue. One theory is that BPH is an immune-mediated inflammatory disorder (Mills & Bone, 2013). There is an inverse relationship between testosterone and inflammatory markers, such as the inflammatory cytokines: Il6, TNF-alpha, Il beta (Maggio et al., 2015). Low testosterone levels are also related to low cortisol levels or cortisol resistance, which again relates to inflammation and fatigue factors. It has been suggested that men harbour their concerns in their prostate and this may be a portal for the expression of endogenous heat issues, especially where these are related to personal relationships and intimacy.

There is a relationship between low testosterone levels and metabolic syndrome. Metabolic syndrome is a combination of hypertension, truncal weight gain, type 2 diabetes and hypercholesterinaemia which carries a high risk of cardiovascular incidence. Metabolic syndrome is a consequence of adrenal dysfunction and cortisol deficiency or resistance. Testosterone also directly affects adipose tissue and glucose and lipid metabolism.

Symptoms of prostate dysfunction are generally due to tissue restriction, but this is complicated by the effects of changes in autonomic regulation. Passive sympathetic deficiency causes an increase in parasympathetic activation, which affects smooth muscle tonicity. Urinary tract activity is increased with increased micturition, nocturia and changes in flow dynamics. Symptoms may therefore be from a combination of autonomic changes and hormone deficiency, but both are related to problems with fatigue or foundational energy.

Nutritional and lifestyle advice for prostate health	
Anti-inflammatory diet	Avoid red meat, dairy foods, eggs and poultry, processed foods and sugar, alcohol, caffeine.
Low carbohydrate diet	Especially refined carbohydrates.
Avoid acrylamide	Found in many fried foods. Is carcinogenic.
Nuts and seeds	Pumpkin seeds and sesame seeds are especially high in zinc. Zinc is found in high concentrations in the prostate and is thought to help balance testosterone and DHT. Brazil nuts contain selenium. They also contain vitamin E and essential fatty acids.
Tomatoes	Especially cooked are a good source of lycopene, an antioxidant with specific actions on the prostate. Avoid tinned tomatoes as tin cans are lined with bisphenol-A (BPA), a synthetic oestrogen.
Fish	Cold water, oily fish, e.g. salmon, trout, sardines. Rich in omega 3 fatty acids.
Berries	All dark and colourful fruits.
Broccoli	Broccoli and other cruciferous vegetables, including bok choy, cauliflower, Brussels sprouts and cabbage, contain a chemical known as sulforaphane. This is thought to target cancer cells and promote a healthy prostate.

(Continued)

Nutritional and lifestyle advice for prostate health

Vitamin C	Citrus fruits—oranges, lemons, limes and grapefruits are all particularly high in vitamin C and bioflavonoids.
Onions and garlic	
Supplementation	Where the diet is inadequate supplement with: Vitamin D: 3,000 i.u. Vitamin A: 25,000 i.u. Vitamin E: 1,200 i.u. Vitamin C with bioflavonoids: 1,000 mg. Lycopene: 10 mg. Zinc: 15 mg.
Exercise	Raises the sympathetic tone and therefore reduces visceral hyperactivity and congestion and improves the circulation and immune system. Kegel exercises improve circulation to the prostate. Raise the pelvic floor for ten repetitions several times daily.

Herbs for the male reproductive system

(See also herbs for the urinary system)

	Actions	*Applications*
Epimedium	Endocrine tonic and agent, specifically testosterone (Yance, 2013).	Loss of libido. Prevents negative effects of cortisol. Prostate cancer.
Equisetum	Haemostatic. Astringent.	Prostatitis. Cystitis. Urethritis. Enuresis.
Hydrangea arborescens	Stimulating and relaxing diuretic. Anti-inflammatory for the urinary tract and prostate (Ross, 2010).	Prostatitis. Urinary tract inflammation and pain, urinary difficulty, calculi. BPH.
Serenoa	Restoring, pungent, astringent, sweet. Endocrine tonic. Genitourinary tonic and alterative. Diuretic, urinary antiseptic. Endocrine stimulant. Antispasmodic, sedative Expectorant, anti-inflammatory. Depurative.	Male and female sterility, impotence and sexual dysfunction. Gentio-urinary tract infection—PID, ovaritis, salpingitis, orchitis, epididymitis, prostatitis, cystitis. Prostatic hypertrophy, carcinoma. Uterine enlargement. Underdeveloped breast development. PCOS. **Special features: a stimulating depurative tonic for the male and female reproductive and urinary systems for deficiency, congestion and infection.**

(Continued)

	Actions	Applications
		For infertility and deficient sexual activity and development in both sexes. Serenoa decreases the production of DHT from testosterone.
Tribulus	Aphrodisiac, tonic and anti-inflammatory. Stimulates testosterone and DHEA production (Yance, 2013).	Impotence, low libido, male infertility.
Trigonella	Aromatic, warming, demulcent.	Warming nourishing tonic for sexual debility (Ross, 2010).
Turnera diffusa	Stimulating, restoring, bitter, pungent. CNS stimulant. Aphrodisiac. Nerve trophorestorative, thymoleptic. Diuretic. Laxative.	Stimulant to the digestive tract—dyspepsia, constipation. Enuresis, irritable bladder. Prostatic hypertrophy. Amenorrhoea, dysmenorrhoea. Premature ejaculation and sexual weakness. **Special features: stimulating tonic, restorative and balancer for the CNS and ANS in depressed, debilitated and deficient conditions and with particular connection to the generative system. Impotence, sexual deficiency and sexual dysfunction in both sexes.**
Urtica radix	Diuretic. Restorative tonic for the kidneys, bladder and prostate.	Specific for BPH. Prostate cancer inhibitor.

Case history: benign prostatic hypertrophy

This man, aged 65, has been experiencing the symptoms of BPH for some four or five years, which have slowly worsened. The diagnosis of the GP has been confirmed by a consultant. The main symptoms are an impaired urinary flow and some difficulty starting and stopping. He has nocturia one or two times per night. He describes his libido as poor and ejaculation as absent. His prostate-specific antigen (PSA) has been measured at a consistent 0.9. He took Saw Palmetto in capsule form for some time, which improved his urinary flow but reduced his libido.

He describes his energy and vitality as good and he has no other significant health problems. He is of normal weight, well dressed, sociable and articulate.

Clinical signs:
Blood pressure: 146/90.
Pulse: 52.

Pulse pressure: 56.
Tongue: slightly swollen, dry and with anterior heat.

Analysis and interpretation:
There would appear to be some prostatic impediment to urinary flow, although it is difficult to separate this from changes in smooth muscle tonicity as a consequence of changes in the autonomic system, e.g. in this case, slightly raised diastolic tension in the circulation, which subsequently decreased. The key factor is endocrine depletion and reduced testosterone levels. The tongue shows some endogenous heat and there is the possibility of some inflammatory factors.

Rationale:
The formulation is designed to nourish and restore the endocrine system, both in general and in the promotion of testosterone production.

Herb	Dosage	Actions
Panax ginseng	30.00	Endocrine agent, tonic/restorative.
Centella asiactica	20.00	Tonic, anti-inflammatory.
Schizandra chinensis	10.00	Activating, warming, dispersing tonic.
Trigonella foenum-grecum	20.00	Aromatic, warming, demulcent and nourishing tonic for sexual debility.
Serenoa repens	30.00	Endocrine tonic and stimulant, genitourinary tonic and alterative.
Urtica officinale radix	30.00	Genitourinary tonic and restorative.
Polygonum multiflorum	20.00	Restorative and nitrifying endocrine agent.
Hydrangea arborescens	15.00	Genitourinary anti-inflammatory.
Epimediium saggitatum	30.00	Anabolic agent and endocrine tonic.
	205.00	

Three months:
Blood pressure: 130/80.
Pulse: 50.
Pulse pressure: 50.

Urinary flow improved. Nocturia absent or once per night. Libido improved and ejaculate has some fluid. Energy generally has improved.

Case history: prostate cancer 1

This professional artist, aged 76, has prostate cancer. This man sought medical assistant after experiencing frequency and urgency of micturition and a slow flow. He has nocturia usually twice nightly. He reports his energy and well-being as good, 8 or 9/10.

Clinical signs:
Blood pressure: 138/80.
Pulse: 88.
Pulse pressure: 58.

Medical tests:
PSA: 4.8, previously 8.1.
Gleeson scale 6.
Biopsy and MRI reveal a nodular cancer.
Takes zinc and selenium.

Centella 15
Panax. 20
Curcuma 20
Larrea. 15
Rhodiola 15
Calendula 15
Serenoa 30
Hydrangea 15
Zanthoxylum 5
Dosage: 5 ml bid aq ac.

Case history: prostate cancer 2

This man of 64 was diagnosed with prostate cancer following a routine blood test, which revealed an elevated PSA. Biopsy revealed 2 out 12 positive and rated 6/10. Reported as slow growing and relatively stable. Monitoring protocol: Blood tests for PSA every 3 months and MRI/biopsy every 12 months.

Clinical signs:
Blood pressure: 146/84.
Tongue: swollen, clear
Zinc taste test negative.

Fruitforce two time daily
Selenium
Biotin
Vitamin B complex
Saw palmetto

Three years:
Blood pressure: 120/76.
Prostate symptoms NAD.

Centella. 30
Astragalus. 30
Schizandra. 15
Hydrastis 15
Urtica radix. 20
Hydrangea. 20
Rosmarinus. 20
Dosage: 5 ml bid aq ac.

The thyroid

Hypothyroidism

Hypothyroidism is indicative of a repressed, deficient and congested response. Secondary hypothyroidism is probably very underdiagnosed, and there are many subclinical cases that are related to fatigue syndrome. In adrenal fatigue, the body may seek to reduce functionality in order to preserve resources, and one way of achieving this is to reduce the metabolic rate by reducing thyroxine output. Low body temperature, especially on rising, reduced pulse rate and a tendency to gain weight easily may be indications of subclinical hypothyroidism dependent upon a fatigue syndrome.

Testing for thyroid function is often minimal. Hypothyroidism from any cause is treated with replacement and so there is little incentive to test for anti-thyroid peroxidase or anti-thyroglobulin. Frequently, only TSH is tested and this can be very unreliable as an indicator of thyroid activity.

Hyperthyroidism

Hyperthyroidism is indicative of hyperactivity, hysteria and lack of control and regulation. Secondary hyperthyroidism may follow periods of stress, overwork and over-striving and is particularly prevalent at times of significant hormonal change, e.g. the menopause and post-partum.

Grave's disease is an inflammatory, autoimmune condition that produces a secretory multinodular goitre with hypersecretion of thyroxine.

Nutrition

Treatment protocols often emphasise the importance of iodine, which can be extremely important, but deficiency is not inevitable and supplementation when not indicated is counterproductive. Iodine deficiency may be an issue due to competitive inhibition from other halogens, i.e. fluoride and chlorine. Zinc, magnesium and B vitamins are essential; selenium is important to the activation of triiodothyronine (T3). Kelp (Laminaria) and other sea foods, are a rich source of iodine and other minerals. It should be noted, however, that sea products can be contaminated with heavy metals to which the thyroid is very sensitive.

Primary hypothyroidism may have a number of causes; genetic, iodine deficiency goitre, iatrogenic, e.g. lithium. Many cases are however inflammatory in nature and regarded as auto-immune thyroiditis, e.g. Hashimoto's. Thyroiditis is connected with endogenous heat and there is almost invariably a history of sore throat or tonsillitis. Chronic tracking of a heat syndrome to the throat is a pernicious factor. Primary and secondary hypothyroidism are not mutually exclusive and could be expected to co-exist. A fatigue syndrome would be expected to create a deficiency profile, which in turn would tend to exacerbate a heat problem by compression or internalisation and creating aggravation. It is not coincidental that Hashimoto's often develops in the 40s age group, when the capacity to compensate for energy depletion is diminished and life events become problematical.

Thyroid tonics.	Fucus: actions go beyond the source of iodine and minerals. Withania.
Tonics for endocrine support. Actions through the adrenals, pituitary or hypothalamus.	Panax ginseng. Eleutherococcus senticosis. Polygonum multiflorum. Centella asiatica. Salvia officinalis. Rosmarinus officinalis. Smilax officinalis. Urtica (seed).
Regulation of pituitary function.	Vitex agnus castus.
Heat syndrome.	Iris versicolor. Carbenia benefictus. Artemisia spp.
Activation.	Rhodiola rosea. Withania sominera. Selenium.
Hyperthyroid regulation.	Lycopus europaeus/virginicus—decreases T4 to T3 conversions, reduces cardiovascular overactivity. Melissa officinalis—affects TSH action, carminative and spasmolytic. Stachys sylvatica.
Hyperthyroid symptoms. To reduce cardiovascular overactivity, tachycardia, palpitations.	Leonorus cardiaca. Crataegus spp. Viscum alba. Lycopus spp.

Case history: primary hypothyroidism

Significant weight gain (unrelated to dietary intake). Fatigue. Inclination to heat and hot sweats at night.

The 43-year-old patient presented with a diagnosis of primary hypothyroidism following a routine blood test and is being offered levothyroxine as a treatment strategy. She is adamant that she doesn't wish to take hormone replacement and is seeking a natural solution. There is no information available on immunological dysfunction.

The patient has endeavoured to correct her weight gain by undertaking heroic episodes of exercise despite often feeling exhausted.

	0	4 months	6 months	7 months	12 months	18 months
TSH (0.3–5.5)	11.5	4.66	67.9	67.5	90.5	3.25
T4 (12–20)	10.8		5.3	5.3	4.1	
BP	128/80					
Pulse	68					
PP	48					

Clinical signs (aged 18):
Blood pressure: 126/65.
Pulse: 88.
Tongue: red base, red papillae in the tip, slight white coating.

Clinical interpretation and analysis:

Fatigue syndrome—adrenal fatigue associated with lowered thyroid function. Deficiency leads to internalisation of heat.

Liver heat syndrome. Related historically to sore throats and tonsillitis. Endogenous heat tracks to the throat and may be associated with unexpressed emotion.

Immunological autoimmune response. It is an informed judgement that this is a case of thyroiditis, e.g. Hashimoto's.

Herb	Dosage	Actions	Energetic actions
Achillea millefolium	15.00	Stimulating circulatory tonic.	Circulatory regulator.
Centella asiatica	20.00	Adaptogen. CNS and ANS regulator. Anti-inflammatory. Anxiolytic and antidepressant (Gohil et al., 2010). Thyroid stimulant (Gupta et al., 2016).	ANS regulator.
Panax ginseng	20.00	Adaptogen. Tonic.	Foundation tonic.
Schizandra chinensis	10.00	Adaptogen.	Regulation of 'fire'. Adjunct for tonic actions.

(Continued)

Herb	Dosage	Actions	Energetic actions
Iris versicolor	15.00	Bitter. Lymphatic. Hepatic.	Specific for liver heat resolution.
Withania somnifera	15.00	Adaptogen. Endocrine agent. Amphoteric on thyroid function.	Specific for frenetic, chaotic conditions.
Polygonum multiflorum	30.00	Adaptogen. Endocrine restorative.	Foundational substrate tonic.
Rhodiola rosea	15.00	Adaptogen. Nervine. Immune stimulant.	Activating tonic.
Salvia triloba	10.00	ANS regulator.	Engenders sense of self and self-regulation.
Dosage: 5 ml bid aq ac	150.00		

Therapeutic considerations:

- A diet low in inflammatory foods
- Gentle to moderate, enjoyable exercise and no extreme exercise
- Iodine deficiency (seek medical testing to check)
- Iodine deficiency through competitive inhibition from other halogens, e.g. fluorine
- Vitamin and mineral deficiencies: vitamin D, magnesium, selenium

Case history: hyperthyroidism

Presenting complaint

Hyperthyroidism has been diagnosed for four years. She has thyroid nodules. She has been offered a choice of treatment of radioactive iodine or surgery and she is keen to avoid either. She has been experiencing severe migraine for two years. These last for up to two days and are very debilitating. Their frequency has reduced but they now last longer. They tend to be hormone related. She feels disconnected.

She feels she has lots of energy. She is very hot and takes a high fluid intake. She has frequent palpitations.

MC: irregular and heavy but has become normalised through taking nutritional supplements.

This 38-year-old lady is tall and lean and appears well dressed and groomed. She is clearly hot. Her neck is visibly swollen and nodular. She is articulate and sociable. She is in a long-term and happy relationship. She thinks that her thyroid became a problem following a number of stressful events including the tragic death of a close personal friend.

Clinical signs:
Blood pressure: 122/82.
Pulse: 92.
Pulse pressure: 60.
Tongue: swollen, red with a significant central fissure.

Herb	Dosage	Actions
Centella asiatica	20.00	CNS/ANS regulator. Anti-inflammatory.
Smilax officinalis	20.00	Foundational tonic and restorative. Anti-inflammatory.
Schizandra chinensis	10.00	Adjunct for tonics.
Taraxacum officinalis radix	15.00	Foundational and grounding tonic.
Lycopus europaeus	15.00	Thyroid regulator. Cardiovascular sedative.
Stachys betonica	20.00	Cerebral-spinal restorative and nervine tonic.
Borago officinalis	25.00	Adrenal cortical tonic.
Rosmarinus officinalis	15.00	Autonomic regulator.
Ocimum santum	10.00	Aromatic and resolving agent.
	150.00	

Flower essences:
Agrimony
Sob
Rock Rose
Cherry Plum
Walnut
Tr Prunella vulgaris 7ggt

Clinical signs progression

	0 weeks	2 weeks	6 weeks	12 weeks
BP	122/82	118/80	118/80	114/64
Pulse	92	94	76	74
PP	40	38	38	50
CVI	18,768	18,612	15,048	13,172
Tongue	Swollen red base.	Reduced heat.		
Symptoms		Feeling generally better.	Feeling generally better. Three times palpitations. Two times migraines.	Occasional headache. Neck shows no nodules.

The muscular-skeletal system

> The truth shall make you free, but first it shall make you angry.
>
> (Unknown)

> Holding on to anger is like grasping a hot coal with the intent of throwing it at someone else; you are the one who gets burned.
>
> (Buddha)

Chronic inflammatory conditions are a complex combination of different factors, which may affect one or more of the organ systems as well as the muscular-skeletal system, and their aetiology is complex. Inflammation is probably associated with most, if not all, chronic disease processes, but is not necessarily recognised. Inflammation is a tissue-based immunological mechanism, which is identified by specific diagnostic tests. What isn't clear is the role played by less embedded immunological mechanisms, i.e. endogenous heat. Heat is evidenced by signs and symptoms but is not necessarily identifiable from clinical tests. Heat as an aetiological factor in muscular-skeletal conditions, and in fact any chronic disease process, and is clearly a key immunological issue, but not one that is recognised in orthodox medicine.

Rheumatoid arthritis would be diagnosed as an inflammatory disease on the basis of tests for inflammation, whereas osteoarthritis, which lacks the inflammatory markers, is labelled as a disease process of wear and tear. It has been more recently accepted, however, that osteoarthritis inevitably involves an element of inflammation alongside changes in anabolic metabolism associated with endocrine depletion and other factors. The influence of heat factors is identifiable in many conditions by examination of the timeline of the development of a pathology. An older person with chronic and progressive osteoarthritis may well demonstrate a history of sore throats and tonsillitis in childhood and, for example, migraine in their young adult life. This demonstrates the expression of a heat condition through different portals, which change according to the circumstances of the physiological balance. Arthritis may be a late manifestation of a heat condition, which has been through a number of representations. Arthritis is a deeper condition of heat as it is expressed in the joints and connective tissues, thus presenting a more somatised problem. It is further complicated by the endocrine changes that occur with age, in particular adrenal cortical depletion and the reduction in cortisol production. Cortisol is the key regulator of inflammation. Heat in the general sense is related to the development of inflammation but can be regarded as a psycho-physiological immunological expression of repressed emotion.

The neural pathways for the experience of emotional pain are the same as those as for physical pain, involving the anterior insula and the anterior cingulate cortices. Most of the processing of pain is in the brain, although the experience is in the part of the body affected. The anterior cingulate is located anatomically closely with the premotor cortex, and so emotional pain has a direct connection with physicality and movement. Unexpressed emotion, such as anger, can result in muscular tension and strain, which is a reflex of the emotional constraint involved. Physical pain and symptoms can therefore give a direct perception of the emotional state that underlies it. The connection between emotion and physicality are commonly linked in language, e.g. 'pain in the neck', 'they make me feel sick' (Fogel, 2013).

Factors associated with inflammation

Changes in the circulatory dynamics
The balance of the autonomic nervous system is key to inflammation. Sympathetic deficiency and parasympathetic excess directly increase the inflammatory and pain responses. Agents that improve the autonomic balance automatically improve pain and inflammation. Sympathetic deficiency may be active or passive, or more likely a combination of both. Deficiency directly affects the internalisation of heat.

Depletion of vitality
Endocrine imbalance through depletion factors, menopause etc., affect the vital response and the capacity to provide compensatory mechanisms. For example, adrenal fatigue and low cortisol or cortisol resistance allow for an uncontrolled inflammatory response.

Autoimmune reactions
Inflammatory reactions to body tissues possibly as a consequence of sensitisation by pathogens, toxins, or allergy. In herbal therapeutic terms it is a further internalisation of endogenous heat.

Congestion
Congestion is an inevitable element of inflammation and may be aggravated by toxin release by acute, chronic or subclinical infection or allergic reactions. Congestion requires the use of herbal agents to clear the tissues.

(Continued)

Factors associated with inflammation (continued)

Relationship to chronic emotional disturbance
The timeline and circumstances of the condition will normally provide insight into the aetiological emotional factors involved, e.g. shock, grief, anger and depression. There may be links to abuse in all of its forms. Abuse often leads, not only to emotional repression, but to the lack of development of personal authority and the capacity for effective decision-making and the ability for controlling the personal psycho-social environment.

Exogenous pathogenic influences
Cold, damp, wind and heat can be aggravating factors when the vital response and compensatory mechanisms are compromised. For example, arthritis often shows dramatic improvement in a warm, dry environment.

Chronic infection
Chronic infection is associated with a high proportion of inflammatory conditions, although the relationship with causality is not always clear. Viruses in the herpes group, e.g. Epstein Barr, are often implicated.

Factors to improve inflammation

Calorie load
A high calorie diet and obesity aggravate inflammation. A low calorie, or preferably, a ketogenic diet is essential.

Exercise
Regular, gentle exercise is essential. This promotes sympathetic activation, the vital response and improves the circulatory dynamics. Exhaustive exercise is damaging and may be a key factor in the development of inflammation.

Sleep
Good sleep is essential for restoration. Melatonin production, associated with good sleep, is directly related to thymus activity and immune modulation.

Nutrition
A diet rich in fruit and vegetables, not only for nutrient content but also for anti-oxidants. Check for food allergies and sensitivities.
Omega 3 fatty acids (arachidonic acid is an omega 6 fatty acid that causes a pro-inflammatory hormone response, eicosapentaenoic acid is omega 3 fatty acid that is anti-inflammatory).
Vitamin D is essential not only for calcium metabolism but also for its anti-inflammatory and immune modulating actions.

Herbal actions

Anti-inflammatories The action of some herbal anti-inflammatories is complex and is not necessarily purely symptomatic; some are also depurative and protective in action.	Harpagophytum procumbens. Menyanthes trifoliate. Guaiacum officinalis. Salix alba. Filipendula ulmaria. Calendula officinalis. Chamomilla spp. Fraxinus excelsior. Populus spp. Tanacetum parthenium.

(Continued)

Herbal actions (continued)

Herbs with hormonal and anti-inflammatory actions.	Dioscorea villosa. Cimicifuga racemose. Angelica sinensis.
Tonics To lend support, structure and balance to the vital organs and overall vitality, i.e. in degenerative conditions there is an emphasis upon catabolism and a deficiency in anabolism, which leads to tissue disintegration. Many are directly anti-inflammatory.	Smilax officinalis. Centella asiatica. Panax ginseng. Borago officinale. Polygonum multiflorum.
Diaphoretic and circulating herbs Important to improve circulatory dynamics and create a constructive tone. Constriction may be non-specific, e.g. created by sympathetic deficiency or specific and related to trauma, e.g. shock.	Achillea millefolium. Angelica archangelica. Anenome pulsatilla.
Depuratives Important to act upon toxic heat but require careful use to avoid worsening the situation or creating difficult cleansing reactions.	Liver and kidney herbs. Taraxacum officinale. Arctium lappa (radix and seed). Galium aparaine. Rumex crispus.
Demulcents and tissue healing herbs to heal, restore and tone tissue.	Althaea officinalis. Plantago spp. Petroselinum crispum. Symphytum officinale. Agropyron repens.
Topical applications—counter irritants, volatile oil. There are different schools of thought on the use of hot v cold treatments for inflamed tissues.	

Pathology

Arthritis

- Osteoarthritis
- Rheumatoid
- Gout
- Inflammatory

Osteoporosis

- Frozen shoulder
- Fibrositis

- Polymyalgia rheumatica
- Carpal tunnel syndrome
- Tenosynovitis
- Dupuytrens contracture
- Hallux rigidus

Herbs for the muscular-skeletal system

Corydalis spp.	Anodyne. Anti-inflammatory. Spasmolytic.	Chronic inflammatory conditions, especially arthritis. Dysmenorrhoea.	In Chinese medicine Corydalis is used as a kidney tonic, fitting for an anti-inflammatory herb associated with adrenal depletion.
Guaiacum off. Constituents: Resins. Phenolic lignans. Terpenoids. Cautions: avoid in acute inflammation of the digestive tract. Combinations: Smilax, Curcuma, Hydrastis. Dosage: Tr 1:5—1–4 ml.	Anti-inflammatory Depurative. Circulatory stimulant. Astringent. Diuretic. Laxative. Expectorant.	Chronic skin conditions—psoriasis, furunculosis, eczema, abscess. Joint conditions—rheumatoid, toxic, osteo-arthritis, gout. Chronic pulmonary conditions—chronic bronchitis, congestion. Dupuytrens contracture. Tonsillitis. Mercurial poisoning. Amenorrhoea and dysmenorrhoea.	A stimulating depurative for all conditions of toxic heat and inflammation with particular reference to the skin and joints. Specific to detoxify the system of mercury.
Harpagophytum procumbens Constituents: Iridoid glycosides, phenols, amino acids, sterols, triterpenes. Cautions: Pregnancy, peptic ulceration. Dosage: Tr 1:5—< 5 ml capsule or tablet 250 mg 2–3 times daily.	Anti-inflammatory. Bitter tonic, hepatic, cholagogue. Lymphatic. Cholesterol reducing. Diuretic. Analgesic, sedative. Antipyretic.	Musculoskeletal pain and inflammation—arthritis, fibromyalgia, fibrositis, sciatica, lumbago. Digestive stimulant—dyspepsia, heartburn, flatulence. Hypercholesteraemia, arteriosclerosis. Hepatic congestion. Pruritis, acne, psoriasis. Furunculosis.	Cleansing and anti-inflammatory action for all conditions of toxic and inflammation reactions affecting the joints, GIT or GUT.

(Continued)

Menyanthes trifoliate	Anti-inflammatory.	Musculoskeletal pain	A stimulating
Constituents:	Depurative.	and inflammation—	depurative with
Iridoid glycosides.	Tonic.	rheumatism, myalgia.	particular effect on
Pyridine alkaloids.	Diuretic.	Digestive stimulant	the liver, lymphatics
Flavanol glycosides.	Astringent.	and tonic—	and digestive
Steroids, volatile	Choleretic.	anorexia, dyspepsia,	function, for all
oils, coumarins,	Analgesic.	constipation.	conditions of toxic
terpenoids, tannin.		Hepatic congestion.	and inflammatory
Cautions: acute			muscular-skeletal
inflammatory			complaints.
conditions of the GIT.			Migraine of hepatic
Combinations:			origin.
Apium.			Decongesting
Dosage:			for constricted
Tr 1:5—0.5–2 ml.			hot conditions
			associated with the
			liver and digestive
			tract.

Case history: fibromyalgia

This lady, aged 62, complains of significant fatigue, especially upon rising in the mornings and in the evenings. She has muscular aches and pains especially in her limbs, these are always present but vary in intensity due to fatigue, stress and changes in the weather. Her head is generally clear with good focus and concentration when she is at work but when not at work she is muzzy-headed and disorientated. She has significant and deep-seated kidney ache.

This lady has had a very stressful history. She was a refugee from the Croatian War of Independence, having experienced significant shock and turbulence. Her first husband died, leaving her with a daughter. Of particular tragedy was the death of her sister at the age of 23, from leukaemia, which has left a lasting imprint of grief. In recent years she has nursed her ageing parents until their deaths.

Clinical signs:
Blood pressure: 130/80.
Pulse: 62. Pulse character: deep and empty.
Pulse pressure: 50.
Tongue: pale and swollen, heat to the tip and edges.

Self-prescribed supplements: vitamin D, turmeric, magnesium, calcium, 5HTP, and black cherry extract.

The patient has an encouraging prognosis as she is employed in a technically challenging and lucrative occupation and is desperate to sort out her health problems. This would suggest that she does not have any significant investment in her health problems, i.e. primary or secondary gain. She has been prescribed a number of orthodox medications, which she now refuses to take as they are ineffective and have troublesome side effects.

Her symptoms and clinical signs suggest that her energy profile is reflective of her need for effective engagement, i.e. her sympathetic output is compatible with the demands of work but is deficient when not at work. So, generally, she is not deficient but probably has a considerable degree of depletion against which she has to exert herself. Her pulse rate is relatively slow and would suggest a slow metabolism, the most likely cause of which would be hypothyroidism, either clinically or sub-clinically. The character of the pulse is deep and empty, suggesting that her endocrine system is struggling to maintain sympathetic output. The heat in the tongue is indicative of an endogenous heat pattern and there are no blood test results to indicate whether this is measurable inflammation. The heat may be a combination of active and positive elements. Active in the sense that it relates to unresolved emotional trauma and passive in the sense that there is dysregulation of the control mechanism of inflammatory response, i.e. cortisol deficiency from depletion factors.

A key factor in her situation may be an impairment in her capacity to implement effective decision-making in terms of care of herself. This is a contradiction to her obvious capacity for decision-making in her occupation and external life. This is often the consequence of being raised in an environment of compliance with adult authority and may lead to entering controlling relationships. Her relationship with her husband is strained. He is retired but makes no contribution to domesticity at all and has no interest or commitment to her health and well-being.

Agreed therapeutic aims:

- Nourishment of foundational energy
- Embodiment
- Release (from a sense of restraint)

Herb	Physiological actions	Energetic actions
Angelica archangelica radix	Spasmolytic. Stimulating and relaxing.	Protective. Sense of calm and peace.
Centella asiatica	Adaptogen. CNS and ANS regulator. Anti-inflammatory. Anxiolytic and antidepressant (Gohil et al., 2010).	ANS Regulator.
Smilax	Foundational tonic and adaptogenic. Anti-inflammatory.	Sense of authority. Foundation.
Schizandra chinensis	Adjunct for tonic actions.	Regulation of the 'fire' principle.

(Continued)

Herb	Physiological actions	Energetic actions
Agrimonia	Stabilising physiologically and psychologically.	Resolution of liver endogenous heat.
Borago	Adrenal tonification.	Courage and resolve.
Stachys betonica	Cerebral-spinal regulator. Nerve tonic.	Autonomic regulation of the psycho-social interconnection.
Verbena officinale	Nerve tonic and restorative.	Self-affirmation and strength.
Salvia triloba	ANS regulator.	Engenders sense of individuation and self-regulation.
Agrimony Walnut Elm Star of Bethlehem Cherry Plum Olive	Acceptance. Protection from outside influence. Trust. Forbearance. Shock.	

Additions after two months

Taraxacum officinale	Foundational tonic. Depurative.	Embodiment and self-connection. Growth.
Chanomeles	Neuromuscular connection.	

The patient showed a steady improvement in symptoms. Interestingly after a period of approximately three months her husband demanded a divorce, to which she readily agreed. Subsequently the house was sold and she bought an attractive property at a good price, which she really loves. She has developed her own independent lifestyle.

Changes in blood pressure:

- One month: Blood pressure: 136/78. Pulse: 66.
- Two months: Blood pressure: 124/70. Pulse: 66.
- Three months: Blood pressure: 102/62. Pulse: 76.
- Four months: Blood pressure: 122/70. Pulse: 72.

One year:
Blood pressure: 124/70.
Pulse: 66.
Pulse pressure: 54.
Much reduced heat in the tongue.

Generally feeling calm and balanced. Little muscular aches and pains. Reduced but continuing problem with phlegm.

The resolution of emotional conflict is difficult to milestone being due to a complex milieu of acceptance, personal growth and authentication, self-belief and self-actualisation, i.e. is a process through which one progresses. She certainly feels much improvement in terms of mental and emotional well-being and mood. She has noticed an enhanced interest in colour, flowers and other natural things, i.e. an enhancement in sensorial appreciation.

The patient requested additional help with the phlegm and a new formula was designed. The phlegm would appear to be a deeper issue, which predated her other health problems and is lifelong.

Herb	Physiological actions	Energetic actions
Achillea millefolium		
Astragalus	Tonic and adaptogen specifically for the immune system.	Sense of the capacity to control and regulate one's boundaries.
Schizandra chinensis	Adjunct for tonic actions.	Regulation of 'fire'.
Hydrastis canadenis	Membrane tonic and astringent.	Breaking old unhelpful patterns.
Althaea officinalis radix	Mucous membrane demulcent.	
Thymus serpentina	Tonic, aromatic membrane restorative.	
Petroselinum officinale	Parasympathetic drainer. Anti-allergy. Restorative.	
Rosa damacena	Resolution of heat.	Resolver of emotional negative patterns.
Salvia triloba	ANS regulator.	Engenders sense of individuation and self-regulation.

Two months following the new formula:
Blood pressure: 112/66.
Pulse: 66.
Pulse pressure: 46.

The phlegm was much improved. The patient reported feeling dizzy on occasions. What appeared to become manifest was that she was becoming responsive to her situation; unlike previously when she lived with the experience of a tense charge and her sympathetic output was reduced, more variable, and on occasions deficient. The patient reflected that her fibromyalgia commenced about ten months after she married and disappeared at about the time her husband left.

Case history: arthritis

This 69-year-old woman, complains of significant pain in both of her knees upon exercise. They have been worsening over a period of some six years. A walk of some quarter of a mile becomes very painful. She also has pain on movement in her left shoulder and left ankle. She has some variable lower back pain. Her muscles are generally stiff in the morning and take an hour or two to loosen up. Blood tests are negative for inflammatory markers.

She describes her energy as reasonable but she is not very good first thing in the morning. She describes her mood as generally low and pessimistic. She describes her temperature as generally normal, although she dislikes excess heat. Her peripheral circulation is normal, her head is clear and she does not experience headache. Her digestion is described as normal and she has no apparent problem with any food groups.

This lady is a little reticent and uncertain in manner, but articulate and coherent. She is clearly significantly overweight and looks fatigued.

Orthodox medicine: Dosulepin 25 mg, Beconase nasal spray, Zolpidem.

Previous medical history:
Rheumatic fever age 8. A history of sore throats and tonsillitis.

Clinical signs:
Blood pressure: 120/72.
Pulse: 66.
Pulse pressure: 48.
CVI: 12,672.
Tongue: very swollen, pale, central fissure.

Analysis and interpretation:
It is difficult to determine the weighting of the causative factors of the condition. Mainstream medicine would not consider this to be rheumatoid arthritis, due to the lack of inflammatory markers, and therefore, by default, would diagnose osteoarthritis—usually regarded essentially as a 'wear and tear' problem. However, even in mainstream medicine, there is a movement towards recognising that all forms of arthritis involve some element of inflammation. From the herbal medicine perspective, it would be seen as a development of an endogenous heat problem that had progressed through different guises since childhood and certainly would consider the rheumatic fever and the history of sore throats as significant. The possible reasons pertaining to the development of the heat syndrome were not investigated or discussed. Such a dialogue does not necessarily assist the intervention process and may hinder by invoking a defensive reaction and consequent non-compliance. Interestingly, the heat is now at the level of the connective tissues and there are no signs of heat in terms of more superficial manifestation or in the tongue, therefore the heat could be regarded as a somatised pattern. Similarly, heat is often related to signs of congestion and tension and this patient does not demonstrate such a pattern, having relatively low CVI but evidence of congestion in her tongue. In fact, the clinical signs suggest a slight deficiency, probably due to some endocrine deficiency and depletion factors. The low pulse suggests perhaps a low metabolism and hence low thyroid output.

Treatment intervention:
The intervention provides tonification for the endocrine system and foundation energy. This serves to strengthen the physiological foundation, the patient's inherent personal strength and resolve, and the capacity to move on from the unseen primal influences that burden her. Resolution of the heat pattern is promoted by the combination of Schizandra, Guaiacum, Plantago and Rosa.

Herb	Dosage	Physiological actions	Energetic actions
Centella asiatica	15.00	Tonic/adaptogen. CNS and ANS regulator. Anti-inflammatory.	Central organisation and regulation.
Smilax	30.00	Endocrine tonic and anabolic agent.	Core and foundational strength.
Schizendra chinensis	10.00	Adjunct tonic agent.	Regulation of 'fire'.
Guaiacum	15.00	Anti-inflammatory.	Resolution of deep personal shock.
Plantago lanceolata	15.00	Demulcent and resolvent.	
Rosa damacena	10.00	Liver cooler.	Resolution of heat and emotion.
Polygonum multiflorum	30.00	Endocrine restorative.	
Symphytum herba	20.00	Tissue healing and restorative.	Healing of personal fractures.
Cimicifuga racemosa	15.00	Cerebral-spinal restorative.	

Follow up information

Week	Blood pressure	Pulse	Pulse pressure	CVI	Tongue	Symptoms
0	120/72	55	48	12,672	Swollen, pale.	
4	116/70	68	46	12,648	Less swollen.	Reduced pain, less crunching.
8	116/70	72	46	13,392	Colour improved.	Much less pain, walking without pain, energy improved, cough and cold.

It is interesting to note that at approximately six weeks of treatment, the patient developed a severe cold and consequent cough, following the resolution of this, after approximately two weeks, she noticed a significant general change in her health.

Case history: muscular/skeletal aches and pains

This lady, aged 70, complains of chronic joint pains, and muscle aches, which are of variable and intermittent intensity. Joint pains are mainly to her elbows, wrists, fingers and knees. Muscle aches are mainly to her neck and biceps, but she also has a persistent lower backache. The symptoms are sufficient to be disabling and very distressing and they tend to be worse from mid-afternoon to early evening. She has episodes of intense cold but with occasional hot flushes and antipathy to heat. She had a similar episode seven years previously, the symptoms slowly disappeared but to return severely approximately 3–4 weeks ago. She has significant fatigue, to the point of being unable to fulfil her daily chores effectively, which is much worse when she has worse pain.

Systems:
Digestion: no particular problems apart from a tendency to slight constipation. Reduced appetite.
Micturition: no particular problems.
Cerebral circulation: occasional muzzy heads. Occasional unsteadiness.
Nervous/emotional: she feels emotionally irritable is very dejected about the future.

Clinical signs:
Blood pressure: 98/70.
Pulse: 78.
Pulse pressure: 28.
CVI: 13,104.
Tongue: slight dry, red base, thin white coating.

Context:
This lady is a little overweight, appears pale with a malar flush. She is articulate, sociable and well-groomed. The original symptoms occurred 12 weeks following the death of her husband for whom she was the primary carer. Other significant events are the death of her father 18 months prior to the onset. She remarried approximately five years ago.

This patient has clearly been affected by a number of significant personal challenges, including the classic post-traumatic stress disorder of being a long term carer, with the associated physical and emotional downfall following the death of the cared for, and the associated conflicted emotions experienced. She has significant deficiency and fatigue factors. Following the initial consultation the patient required a hand to steady her when she rose, demonstrating significant orthostatic hypotension. The formulation is a combination of nourishing and regulating tonics to build her foundation, both physiologically and psychologically. Vitamin D and magnesium are essential supplements.

Herb	Dosage	Actions
Angelica sinensis	20.00	Blood tonic and adaptogen.
Centella asiatica	20.00	CNS and ANS regulation and balance. Anti-inflammatory.
Panax ginseng	30.00	Key tonic and adaptogen, personal strength and authority.
Schizandra chinensis	10.00	Adjunct for tonics, regulation of the 'fire' principle.

(*Continued*)

Herb	Dosage	Actions
Guaiacum	10.00	Anti-inflammatory and dispersive.
Glycyrrhiza glabra	15.00	Nutrifying and restorative tonic.
Borago officinalis	20.00	Adrenal tonic and restorative.
Arctium lappa radix	15.00	Restorative tonic for the liver and kidneys.
Eucommia ulmoides	30.00	Endocrine tonic for connective tissues. Strength and flexibility.
Verbena offinale	15.00	
Zingiberis officinalis	5.00	
Flower essences: Olive, Hornbeam, Cherry Plum, Wild Rose, Rock Rose, Agrimony, Star of Bethlehem, Walnut.		To provide: acceptance, trust, balance, protection from intruding influences, release from shock.
Additions: Achillea millefolium	15.00	To improve free circulation.
Salvia officinale	10.00	Hormonal regulation.

Polygonum multiflorum capsules
Magnesium and multivitamin
Vitamin D3

Key actions:
Acceptance, optimism, fortitude, letting go, flexibility, endurance, self-worth.

3 weeks:
The aches/pains and energy improved dramatically but with intermittent poor days. The reappearance of symptoms was generally associated with over exertion and out of the ordinary activities, such as going on holiday. She developed a significant pattern of diarrhoea, which was persistent and didn't respond to intervention or ceasing the Polygonum (aperient action). She was advised to consult a medical diagnosis and a biopsy revealed lymphocytic colitis. This slowly improved without further intervention.

Approximately six months after treatment started she caught a heavy cold and consequently developed a severe and intransigent non-productive cough that improved with medicine.

Herb	Dosage
Angelica arch. Radix	15.00
Centella	15.00
Codonopsis	20.00
Schizandra	10.00

(Continued)

Herb	Dosage
Corydalis	20.00
Tussilago	15.00
Borago	30.00
Hyssopus	15.00
Prunus serotina	15.00

It is suggested that the digestive and respiratory problems that emerged were sequelae to the treatment of a major endogenous heat syndrome. The original consideration was that the heat issues were largely from hormone deficiency, but it would appear that there was probably significantly unresolved emotion.

Twelve months:
Blood pressure: 120/70.
Pulse: 70.
Pulse pressure: 50.
CVI: 13,300.
Tongue, less red (more vibrant pink) little coating.

Energy relatively stable. Aches and pains were occasional and much reduced.

Case history: pain and inflammation

This 65-year-old therapist complains of continuous pain in his left hip following hip replacement therapy three weeks previously. The surgeon is of the opinion that there is no obvious mechanical reason for the pain. The man reports his energy as extremely low.

Clinical signs:
Blood pressure: 98/78.
Pulse: 72.
Pulse pressure: 20 (normal blood pressure 124/78).
Tongue: slightly pale, slight central fissure, central phlegm coating.

Analysis:
The pulse pressure is extremely low and suggests a passive sympathetic deficiency. As a consequence, his pain and inflammatory sensitivity is increased and tissue healing capacity is impaired. The patient knew that he was due to have his hip surgery and made a heroic effort to complete renovations that he had started on his house. Consequently, he entered the surgical procedure in an extremely fatigued state. The strategy is to provide a strong foundational tonic to facilitate the restoration of the sympathetic tone and adrenal cortical function, hence reducing the pain and inflammation and enhancing tissue repair.

Herb	Dosage
Angelica archangelica radix	10.00
Centella asiatica	20.00
Smilax officinalis	20.00
Astragalus membranaceus	15.00
Schizandra chinensis	10.00
Arctium lappa seed	15.00
Polygonum multiflorum	30.00
Borago officinalis	20.00
Rosmarinus officinalis	15.00

Dosage: 5 ml tid aq.

Two weeks:
There was a dramatic improvement in symptom relief and his general energy and vitality. His blood pressure returned to normal levels: 122/78.

Dermatology

Skin pathology may be caused by local conditions, e.g. infection (bacterial, viral, fungal, parasitic), allergy or contact irritation. The majority of serious skin conditions are the manifestation of systemic dysfunction, and treatment should be directed towards the internal disharmony. Conditions are however often multifactorial and complex, with both local and systemic factors playing a part. An allergic response mediated by histamine release may, for example, be amplified by catecholamine stimulation.

There is a close relationship between the skin and the nervous system, both are derived embryologically from the ectoderm. It is apparent that the skin communicates with the nervous system and the nervous system communicates with the skin. The reaction of the ANS to the external environment must influence the neuro-immuno-endocrine response of the skin, as the skin is the crucial barrier protecting the body from the external environment. Most skin conditions arising from constitutional causes are associated with the perception of 'threat' and the consequent reactions of the immune system.

The skin can be important for the expression of emotion, feelings etc., and the distribution of skin problems may be significant. The relationship of skin diseases to the mind and emotions is complex. Some conditions clearly have a strong and direct association, e.g. bullous eczema on the hands, but in many situations the relationship is indirect and relates to organ dysfunction, deficiency and disturbance over a protracted period.

The skin plays an important function in the regulation and protection of the internal environment and as an organ of elimination.

The systemic circulatory dynamics are of paramount importance:

– Congestion in the internal organs causes the retention of heat and toxicity, and problems with metabolism.

– Deficient peripheral circulation results in atrophic conditions of the skin and deficient elimination.

In some circumstances the development of a skin condition may be seen as a superficial manifestation of a deep condition and seen as a good indication following the 'Law of Cure'. Skin conditions are, however, still relatively 'deep' and do not suggest resolution.

The pathology of the skin is involved in a number of deep and intractable conditions regarded as 'autoimmune', e.g. discoid lupus erythematosis, scleroderma, dermatomyositis.

Nutrition

- Vitamins A, B, C, D and E, zinc and selenium, essential fatty acids, bioflavonoids.
- Vitamin D3 is critical in the regulation of inflammation.
- Nutritional status may be important as a secondary action to remedy skin tissue damaged by infection, irritation and inflammation. May also be primary action, i.e. the result of a specific deficiency.

Herbal therapeutic actions

The aetiology of many skin disorders is complex and treatment may necessitate a complex formulation with a number of therapeutic actions. Treatment from the herbal perspective is centred upon the use of depurative herbs. Caution should be observed as depuratives can be powerful and acute symptoms can be made worse and chronic conditions made acute. The use of circulating herbs is often sufficient to initiate a natural cleansing process. A transformative and resolving therapeutic approach is often the best therapeutic intervention.

Depuratives See also hepatics, digestive herbs, astringents, demulcents.	Artium lappa. Taraxacum officinalis radix. Fumaria officinalis. Centaurium erythraea. Scrophularia nodosa. Iris versicolor. Rumex crispus. Trifolium pratense. Viola spp. Urtica diocea. Hydrastis canadensis. Berberis vulgaris, Berberis aquifolium. Lymphatic alteratives—Phytolacca americana. Galium aparine.
Circulating herbs Encourage the movement of energy and blood upwards and outwards in a therapeutic direction. Assist in the balancing of the ANS and CNS.	Achillea millefolium. Angelica spp., Crataegus spp. Tilia spp.
Balancing herbs and tonics Strengthen, support and balance the overall system. Many tonics are also depurative.	Centella asiatica. Smilax officinalis. Schizandra chinensis.

(Continued)

Resolving and transformative.	Aromatics. Lavandula angustifolia, Rosa damascene. Juniperis coomunis. Flower essences.
Anti-inflammatories Useful to control problematical symptoms in the short term. Many are also dupurative and progressive in action.	Guaiacum offinale. Salix alba. Corydalis cava. Chamomilla spp. Calendula officinalis. Arctium lappa seed.
Anti-infectives	Echinacea angustifolia. Thuja occidentalis. Phytolacca Americana. Calendula officinalis. Baptisia tinctoria. Topical—Calendula officinalis. Commiphora molmol. Thuja occidentalis. Lavendula angustifolia. Melaleucca alternifolia.
Topical Treatments Anti-infectives, anti-inflammatories, demulcents, astringents. Careful consideration should made of the suitability of the base used for local applications so as to avoid potential allergic reaction, exacerbate irritation or to create heating actions. Topical applications should be supportive and not suppressive. Topical applications can be treatments as well as providing symptomatic relief.	Calendula officinalis. Stellaria media. Hamamaelis virginiana. Chamomilla spp. Lavendula angustifolia.

Terminology of lesions

Macule A well-defined, flat discolouration of the skin. Redness indicates a vascular source, brown indicates pigmentation, e.g. moles, capillary naevus, freckle, purple staining.

Papule A well-defined, firm elevation of less than 1 cm diameter, e.g. common in eczema, lichen planus, warts.

Plaque A confluence of papules to form an elevated lesion.

Pustule A well-defined projection with a head of pus, which may or may not be septic. Found in the epidermis, hair follicle or sebaceous gland, e.g. acne, bacterial infections.

Vesicle A well-defined projection with a head of serous fluid, a blister.

Bullae Vesicles are <0.5 cm, bullae are larger, e.g. pemphigus, dermatitis herpetiform, acute eczema, burns, herpes.

Scale	A layer of outer epidermis separable from the underlying layer and visible to the naked eye, e.g. psoriasis, ichthyosis.
Erythema	Redness from vascular dilation due to inflammation or nervous reflex. Termed telangiectasia when dilated blood vessels are visible to the naked eye.
Urtica	A weal. A clearly defined raised plateau that develops and disappears rapidly as a consequence of a transient increase in capillary permeability. Has a white or red appearance dependent upon the severity. The weal is surrounded initially by a 'flare'. Usually the result of allergy or hypersensitivity.
Erosion	Damage to the epidermis of mucous membrane as a result of a rupture of a vesicle or bullae.
Ulcer	Damage to the epidermis or dermis, healing results in scarring.
Sclerosis	Hardening of the dermis.
Crust	Dried, coagulated exudate as a result of injury, e.g. weeping eczema, impetigo.

Classification of skin disorders

Eczema

An inflammatory process involving the collection of fluid in the epidermis between the keratinocytes and the upper dermal layer and associated with a perivascular infiltration of lympho-histiolytic cells. The severity of the reaction is expressed in a range of symptoms from acute, associated with bullae to chronic, characterised by thickening, scaling and dryness. It is usually pruritic.

Differentiate between contact dermatitis, allergic dermatitis, atopic eczema and hydriodic or bullous eczema.

Atopic eczema

- Typical of infantile eczema associated with the atopic child and asthma. The typical distribution is to the face and the flexor surfaces of the joints. The appearance may be dryness and thickening of the epidermis through to acute inflammation.
- Associated with IgE mediated immune reaction and lymphocytic infiltration. Milk can be a primary or secondary antigen. Food additives, particularly colours, foods with adrenal-mimetic constituents, e.g. red fruits.
- There is a strong hereditary tendency.
- Constitutionally is associated with 'sensitivity', boundary issues and hyper-parasympathetic tone. There is usually associated vascular constriction, hot/cold issues and behaviour change of hyperactivity or lethargy.
- Secondary complications of bacterial or viral infection are common, e.g. staphylococcus, streptococcus, molluscum.

Discoid

- May be acute or sub-acute. Small lesions widely distributed, particularly on the trunk.
- Often associated with staphylococcus.

Hands

- May be contact or secondary reaction to fungi.
- Bullous or pompholyx may be an acute reaction to stress, particularly in an atopic individual.

Seborrheic

- Inflammation and irritation associated with scaling in hair growing areas, e.g. scalp, axillae, eyebrows, chest.
- Infantile cradle cap and some other instances may relate to an immune response to pityrosporum ovale.
- Other cases can be seen as related to psoriasis.

Venous/varicose

- Usually occurs in older women.
- Often associated with contact dermatitis.
- Associated with venous stasis, hypertension, lymphoedema.

Asteatotic

- The skin of the back of the hands and back has a dry, plate like appearance.
- Often associated with the overuse of soaps and the Winter.
- Common in the elderly due to loss of the stratum cornuem lipids. May have an association with hypothyroidism.

Other pruritic conditions

Pruritis

- Often mediated by histamine, cytokines, tachykinins.
- May relate to anaemia, diabetes, malignancy, renal failure, chronic liver disease, thyroid problems.

Nodular prurigo—itchy papules or nodules on the trunk or extensor surfaces
Lichen simplex—thickened, scaly, hyperpigmentation of the neck, calves, back, genitals.

These conditions are a cutaneous response to scratching or rubbing. Both may co-exist. Typically are more prevalent in the atopic. Often relates to stress.

Psoriasis

Typically manifests as well-defined red scaly plaques and is associated with inflammation and hyperproliferation of the skin. Age incidence occurs in two distributions: 16–22 and 55–60. Incidence is related to infection, e.g. T lymphocyte response to streptococcal infection, drugs, alcohol, stress. Immune complexes are formed to epidermal antigens.

Chronic plaque

- Typically occurs in areas of prolific skin growth, e.g. extensor surfaces but may be extensive. Often starts with a 'herald' patch.
- May be associated with comprised authority issues. Often occurs with reference to relationship problems or shock.
- Flexural.
- Often difficult to diagnose as it does not usually scale and may be confused with tinea.
- Guttate.
- Small eruptions. Often follows approximately two weeks after streptococcal infection and resolves spontaneously after 1–2 months.
- Pustular.

Palmo-plantar psoriasis is confined to the hands and/or feet.

- In extreme form may be related to system symptoms, e.g. malaise, pyrexia, circulatory problems and can be life threatening.
- Psoriasis may also affect the nails or joints.

Psoriasis may be confused with dermatitis herpetiformis, which is associated with gluten enteropathy. The digestive symptoms associated with gluten enteropathy, e.g. bloating and bowel disturbance, may be absent. Psoriasis may also be difficult to distinguish from tinea.

Urticaria

Characterised by itchy weals and swelling. Usually associated with inflammatory mediators, such as histamine.

- Acute episodes usually related to ingestion of an allergen, e.g. seafood, strawberries, drugs or response to a virus or parasite.
- Chronic episodes often related to stress.
- Commoner in the atopic individual.

- Note also: cold urticaria.
- Cholinergic (stress/heat)—small itchy papules on the trunk or arms.
- Dermographia—weals caused by pressure.

Pityriasis rosea

Multiple pink macules usually on the trunk. On the back forms a typical 'Christmas tree' appearance, which follows the nerve distribution. Thought to be a viral rash and resolves spontaneously.

Lichen planus

Presents as small, purple topped polygonal papules, which are intensely itchy. Occurs anywhere, including membranes, but particularly on the flexors of the wrists and lower legs. Lesions may converge into plaques.

Acne vulgaris

Usually starts in adolescence and resolves in adulthood. In females, often relates to the menstrual cycle. Associated with toxic heat conditions and sympathetic deficiency.

Rosacea

Often occurs in later life with individuals who had acne in their teenage years. Involves an element of vasomotor instability in the blood vessels, which may relate to reflex irritation from the upper digestive tract.

Bullous diseases

– Phemigus vulgaris
– Bullous pemphigoid

Dermatitis herpetiformis

Gluten allergy

Linear IgA disease

Associated with autoantibodies binding to the basement membrane, associated with IgA.

Malignant skin tumours

Refer for medical diagnosis and treatment if suspected.

Basal cell carcinomas

Differentiate from a naevus by degree of organisation and blood supply. Not usually invasive. Comprises about 75% of skin cancer.

Squamous cell carcinoma

May spread and metastasise. Related to some kind of trauma to the skin, e.g. sun and may be preceded by solar keratoses. Often occur on the lip, ear or other exposed area. Comprises about 20% of skin cancers.

Malignant melanoma

Usually develop form a pre-existing melanocytic naevi. Often highly invasive and likely to metastasise. Comprises 5% of skin cancers. Often relates to early age sun damage.
Diagnosis strengthened by the following:

- Asymmetry
- Border irregularity
- Colour variation or change
- Diameter >6 mm
- Elevation
- Inflammation
- Bleeding or oozing
- Sensation

Summary of the differential diagnosis of skin conditions:

- Infection—bacterial, viral, fungal
- Classic appearances
- Bacteria—inflammation with pustular or purulent discharge, usually focal, e.g. Streptococcal, staphylococcal
- Viral—bullae
- Fungal—line of inflammation followed by clearance

Inflammatory

- Contact—topical to contact, soap powder
- Response to medicine or food
- Response to substance contact, e.g. IgG inflammatory reaction (linear IgG disease)
- Response to infection—toxic immunological metabolites from infection elsewhere—find focus of infection, e.g. sore throat, often acute rash, e.g. viral

Skin diseases may relate to psychogenic factors, which can be identified from the timeline of the condition and the relationship with critical incidences. There may be an interval of days, weeks, or months between a critical incident and the manifestation of a lesion. Skin disease may be a somatisation of an emotionally distressing event.

Case history: lichen planus

The patient is a 65-year-old housewife who complains of a skin condition that she has had for a period of about four months. The lesions consist of small flat topped polygonal papules on the arms and legs, which are relatively non-pruritic. It started with a 'herald' patch on the left knee and spread along both legs and later to the arms leaving a scar on the areas from which they spread. The doctor has diagnosed infected hair follicles. She describes her general health as very good with no reported problems with energy or well-being.

Clinical signs:
Blood pressure: 140/80.
Pulse: 70.
Pulse pressure: 60.
Tongue: normal colour. Slightly swollen, slight heat papillae in the tip.

This lady has had a trouble-free medical history. She is married with one daughter, now aged 26. She was a late parent, becoming pregnant at the age of 41. This patient describes last year as very stressful due to the death of her younger sister earlier in the year and the poor health of her brother in law. When questioned about her response to her sister's death, she became very emotional. She reports being extremely angry at how the medical profession mistreated her sister.

The formulation is to provide foundation and immunological support and to help the patient move through her grief and anger.

- Angelica archangelica radix
- Centella asiatica
- Arctium lappa semen
- Curcuma longa
- Taraxacum officinalis radix
- Urtica diocea herba
- Verbena officinale
- Viola tricolour
- Rosa damascena

Flower essences: for psycho-spiritual resolution. Acceptance. Letting go.
Rock Rose. Agrimony. Cherry Plum. Star of Bethlehem. Walnut. Holly. Wild Rose.

Follow up:
Blood pressure: 120/70.
Pulse 70.
Pulse pressure: 50.
Tongue: Clear. Slightly swollen.

The skin condition slowly cleared over a period of nine months. The patient decided to reinvent her life and moved with her husband to a fishing village in Scotland where she had spent her honeymoon.

Case history: pompholyx eczema

This retired lady in her 70s presented with pompholyx eczema. Her hands swell and itch followed by itchy vesicles which burst becoming intensely itchy. The skin then becomes dry and flaky. The incidence is episodic, perhaps two or three times per year. No known aggravating factors. Commencement approximately five years previous.

She has a chronic lower back problem (across the lumbar region and into the nerve plexuses), which is aggravated by sitting, relieved by standing and also relieved by sleep, i.e. it improved in the mornings.

Her energy is reported as fine. Digestion is normal but sometimes is bloated after meals. She had surgery for the removal of a duodenal ulcer many years ago and has a stomach of reduced size. She looks frail and older than her years. Her voice is faltering, weak and cracked. Her nails are ridged longitudinally and vertically. She is happily married.

Clinical signs:
Blood pressure: 150/60.
Pulse: 64.
Pulse pressure: 90.
Tongue: slightly swollen with a red, dry and cracked base. Red papillae to the tip. A dry yellow coating over most of the surface.

Context:
Her twin sister died of lung cancer approximately ten years previously and revealed two weeks prior to her death that she had been repeatedly sexually abused by her step-father. This was the same for the patient. The police were reluctant to prosecute. She describes herself as being very angry. She used to avoid him but now confronts him if she meets him. He was also extremely violent. She left home at the age of 19 and never returned, seldom seeing her mother. She is sure that her mother knew of the abuse. She had a younger brother who was the son of the step-father who was killed whilst serving in the army, he left his wife with three young daughters. The step-father used to babysit for the girls and the patient attempted to warn the mother about him.

- Achillea millefolium
- Centella asiatica
- Eucommia ulmoides
- Lycium barbarum
- Plantago lanceolata
- Agrimonia eupatorium
- Corydalis cava
- Arctium lappa seed

- Viola odourata
- Ocimum sanctum
- Citrus aurantium flores

Flower essences: Agrimony, Cherry Plum, Rock Rose, Walnut, Holly.

Follow up:
The skin condition improved over a period of two months and cleared completely. It has not returned over the eight years since treatment.

Case history: chronic urticaria

This professional lady presented with an acute erythematous skin condition to her arms, legs and trunk, which was extremely sore and pruritic, with symptoms presenting for about one week. Her GP practice nurse diagnosed chronic urticaria and prescribed anti-histamines. These were ineffective and the patient was seeking an alternative to steroid treatment. She was extremely distressed and anxious. She has a history of IBS, tension headaches, stress and anxiety, for which she has been treated on a number of occasions.

Context:
This patient has had a very stressful year with problems with a difficult and stressful job and problems with her teenage daughter. There has been a recent improvement in her circumstances and she has recently returned from a two week relaxing holiday during which the symptoms first started (initially she thought it was a food intolerance).

Clinical signs:
Blood pressure: 140/80 (it is normally 128/72).
Pulse: 74.
Tongue: slightly pale, dry and with anterior red papillae.

Herb	Dosage
Centella asiatica	20.00
Panax quinquifolium	20.00
Schizandra chinensis	10.00
Guacicum offinale	15.00
Actium lappa seed	10.00
Plantago lanceolata	30.00
Urtica dioica herba	20.00
Viola odourata	15.00
Ocimum sanctum	10.00

Flower essences: Walnut, Rescue Remedy, Cherry Plum.

During the period of the treatment the patient was told during a visit to a hospital dermatologist that she would never be free of the problem. The patient declined the steroid treatment and continued with the herbal intervention. The condition slowly improved over a six-month period and has been clear ever since. The patient continues with herbal medicine for health promotion.

Case history: herpes simplex

This woman of 23 has had herpes simplex since contracting glandular fever when 16. She usually has two episodes per year, which are very severe and one of these is invariably when on holiday. She develops very itchy and sore blisters on her lips.

She is generally tired, especially in the evenings and very tired when on holiday. She has cold peripheral circulation. Other conditions are mild, chronic asthma, for which she uses an inhaler, and some digestive discomfort and bloating.

Orthodox medicine: contraceptive pill.

Clinical signs:
Blood pressure: 92/60.
Pulse: 56.
Pulse pressure: 32. CVI: 8,512.
Tongue: slight pale, slight dry, anterior heat papillae.
Zinc taste test negative.

The patient has a significant sympathetic deficiency as indicated by the low pulse, low pulse pressure and low systolic blood pressure and this is related to a deficient immunological profile. Significantly, the herpes erupts when on holiday, when she is particularly fatigued and hence deficient. The constitutional medicine is designed to improve her sympathetic tone and provide immunological support. The acute medicine is designed to at work directly on the virus when active.

Constitutional formulation

Herb	Dosage	Actions
Achillea millefolium	15.00	Dispersive circulatory balancer and restorative. Establishment of effective boundaries.
Centella asiatica	15.00	ANS/CNS balancer. Tonic and alterative.
Astragalus membraneous	30.00	Immunological tonic to improve the 'defensive' energy.
Schizandra chinensis	10.00	Tonic adjunct.
Hydrastis canadensis	15.00	Depurative. Resolver of endogenous heat.
Plantago lanceolata	20.00	Demulcent.

(Continued)

Herb	Dosage	Actions
Hypericum plerforatum	20.00	Nervine tonic. Antiviral agent. Liver restorative for liver heat.
Verbena officinalis	15.00	Nervine tonic and restorative.
Lavendula officinalis	10.00	Aromatic and dispersive agent. Antiviral.
Dosage: 5 ml bid.	150.00	

Acute formulation

Herb	Dosage
Achillea millefolium	15.00
Salvia officinalis	10.00
Echinacea angustifolia	30.00
Hydrastis canadensis	15.00
Phytolacca americana	5.00
Hypericum perforatum	20.00
Zingiberis officinalis	5.00
Dosage: 5 ml qid.	100.00

Four weeks:
Blood pressure: 96/60.
Pulse: 64.
CVI: 9984.
Tongue: less pale, less heat.

Case history: eczema

This patient, aged 34, presented with acute eczema to her torso and limbs. It is a lifelong complaint, which she has managed with a variety of creams. The eczema has become much worse over the last six months. She describes her energy as poor but much better when she exercises, which she does on a regular basis. She feels somewhat muzzy and lightheaded. Her menstrual cycle is normally regular and of normal flow but has become irregular over recent months.

This patient is slim, well-groomed, and presented, and is articulate and sociable. She is married with two children.

Clinical signs:
Blood pressure: 110/70.
Pulse: 64.
Pulse pressure: 40.
Tongue: red and very swollen base, deep central flexure, swollen, slippery sides.

Analysis:
Discussion revealed that the patient had taken on a high profile job approximately one year previously. She engaged effectively with the new job and work colleagues in addition to her busy family and personal life but is now experiencing more fatigue and finding life more problematical. The implication is that she raised her sympathetic activation to cope with the increased demands of her work and life and is now experiencing a slight post-traumatic stress disorder and fatigue syndrome. Her clinical signs indicate a degree of sympathetic deficiency, i.e. low pulse pressure. The low pulse is probably indicative of exercise induced cardiac efficiency. The sympathetic deficiency has resulted in fatigue, internalisation of function and compression of systemic heat, hence the eruption of the eczema.

Rationale:
The formulation is composed of three triads. Centella, Astragalus and Schizandra to improve foundational energy, CNS regulation and immunological responsivity. Arctium seed, Rosa and Althaea to resolve the endogenous heat pattern. The Polygonum, Stachys and Verbena to provide autonomic regulation and flexibility, and adaptability of the psycho-social interaction.

Herb	*Dosage*	*Actions*
Centella asiatica	15.00	ANS and CNS regulator.
Astragalus	30.00	Tonic and adaptogen. Immunological balancer and tonic.
Schizandra chinensis	10.00	Tonic adjunct.
Arctium lappa semen	15.00	Stimulating alterative for endogenous heat.
Rosa damascena	10.00	Liver heat resolver.
Althaea officinalis folium	20.00	Demulcent.
Polygonum mutiflorum	20.00	General tonic.
Stachys betonica	20.00	Autonomic balancer and cerebro-spinal restorative.
Verbena officinale	10.00	Nerve tonic and restorative.
Dosage: 5 ml bid aq ac.	150.00	

One month:
Skin completely clear. Energy and well-being improved, head clear.

REFERENCES

Aron, E. (1999). *The Highly Sensitive Child* (Element).
Ball, P. (2006). *The Devil's Doctor* (Arrow Books).
Barker, D. (n.d.). http://www.thebarkertheory.org/ (Accessed on 21 September 2019).
Bartram, T. (1995). *Encyclopedia of Herbal Medicine* (Grace Publishers).
Betterle, C. and Morlin, L. (2011). Autoimmune Addison's disease. In: Ghizzoni, L., Cappa, M., Chrousos, G., Loche, S. and Maghnie, M., eds. *Pediatric Adrenal Diseases. Endocrine Bianchi V. E. Journal of the Endocrine Society*.
Bone, K. and Mills, S. (2013). *Principals and Practice of Phytotherapy Modern Herbal Medicine*, Second Edition (Churchill Livingstone Elsevier).
Braun, C.A. and Anderson, C.M. (2011). *Pathophysiology a Clinical Approach*, Second Edition. (Lippincott Williams and Wilkins).
Bygren, L.O., Kaati, G., Gustafsson, J.A. and Kral, J.G. (2018). Paternal grandparental exposure to crop failure or surfeit during a childhood slow growth period: Epigenetic marks on grandchildren's growth, glucoregulatory and stress genes. Available from https://doi.org/10.1101/215467
Cozolino, L. (2006). *The Neuroscience of Human Relationships* (W.W. Norton).
Cromwell, H.C., Mears, R.P., Wan, L. and Boutros, N.N. (2008). Sensory gating: a translational effort from basic to clinical science. *Clinical EEG and Neuroscience*, 39(2): 69–72.
Daehnert, C. (1998). The false self as a means of disidentification: A psychoanalytic case study. *Contemporary Psychoanalysis*, 34: 251–271.
Denissen, J.J.A., Butalid, L., Penke, L. and van Aken, M.A.G. (2008). The effects of weather on daily mood: A multilevel approach. *Emotion*, 8(5): 662–667.
Dobransky P. (1999). Mind OS: The Operating System of the Human Mind.
Faust, V., Weidmann, M. and Wehner, W. (1974). The influence of meteorological factors on children and youths: A 10% random selection of 16,000 pupils and apprentices of Basle City (Switzerland). *Acta Paedopsychiatrica: International Journal of Child and Adolescent Psychiatry*, 40(4): 150–156.

Fogel, A. (2013). *Body Sense: The Science and Practice of Embodied Self-Awareness* (Norton Series on Interpersonal Neurobiology).

Foucault, M. (1983). *M. Foucault: Beyond Structuralism and Hermeneutics*, 2nd edn, edited by H. Dreyfus and P Rabinow (University of Chicago Press).

Fraiberg, S., Adelson, E. and Shapiro, V. (1975). Ghosts in the Nursery: A Psychoanalytic. Approach to the Problems of Impaired Infant-Mother. *Journal of American Academy of Child Psychiatry*, 14(3): 387–421.

Gohil, K.J. (2010). Pharmacological review on Centella asiatica: a potential herbal cure all. *Indian J Pharm Sci.*, 272(5): 546–556.

Greven, C.U., Lionetti, F., Booth, C., Aron, E.N., Fox, E., Schnedan, H.E., Pluess, M., Bruining, H., Bjittebier, P. and Homberg, J. (2019). Sensory processing sensitivity in the context of environmental sensitivity: A critical review and development of research agenda. *Neuroscience and Biobehavioural Reviews*. Available from https://www.sciencedirect.com/science/article/pii/S0149763418306250?via%3Dihub

Gupta, Y.K., Veerendra Kumar, M.H. and Srivastava A.K. (2003). Effect of Centella asiatica on pentylenetetrazoleinduced kindling, cognition and oxidative stress in rats. *Pharmacol. Biochem. Behav.*, 74: 579–585.

Hardt, J. and Gerbershagen, H.U. (1999). No changes in mood with the seasons: Observations in 3000 chronic pain patients. *Acta Psychiatrica Scandinavica*, 100(4): 288–294.

Hartley, T. (2018). Personal communication.

Hawkes N. (2012). Happiness is a U shaped curve, highest in the teens and 70s, shows survey. *BMJ*, 344, doi: https://doi.org/10.1136/bmj.e1534

Hempton C-H. and Fischer T. (2009). *A Materia Medica for Chinese Medicine* (Churchill Livingstone).

Hippocrates. (400 BCE). On Airs, Waters and Places. Translated by Frances Adams. The Internet Classics Archive. Available from http://classics.mit.edu/Hippocrates/airwatpl.html

Janov, A. (2011). *Life Before Birth* (NTI Upstream).

Janov. A. (1996). *Why You Get Sick and How You Get Well: The Healing Power of Feelings* (Phoenix).

Kaminski, P. and Katz, R. (1994). *Flower Essence Repertory* (The Flower Essence Society).

Kenner, D. and Requena, Y. (1996). *Botanical Medicine: A European Professional Perspective* (Paradigm Publications).

Kolb, B. and Whishaw, I. (2003). *Fundamentals of Human Neuropsychology* (Worth Publishers).

Llewelyn, et al. (2006). *Oxford Hanbook of Clinical Diagnosis* (Oxford University Press).

Longmore, M., Wilkinson, I.B., Baldwin, A. and Wallin, E. (2014). *The Oxford Handbook of Clinical Medicine* (Oxford University Press).

Lowen, A. (1975). *Bioenergetics* (Penguin).

Maciocia G. (2004) *Diagnosis in Chinese Medicine* (Elsevier).

Maggio, M., De Vita, F., Fisichella, A., Lauretani, F., Ticinesi, A., Ceresini, G., Cappola, A., Ferrucci, L. and Ceda, G. (2015). The Role of the Multiple Hormonal Dysregulation in the Onset of "Anemia of Aging": Focus on Testosterone, IGF-1, and Thyroid Hormones. *International Journal of Endocrinology*, pp. 1–22.

Mezzacappa, E.S., Katkin, E.S. and Palmer, S.N. (1999). Epinephrine, arousal, and emotion: A new look at two-factor theory. *Cognition and Emotion*, 13(2): 181–199. Available from doi:10.1080/026999399379320

Miller, A. (1981a). *Thou Shalt Not Be Aware* (Farrar Straus Giroux)

Miller, A. (1981b). *The Drama of the Gifted Child: The Search for the True Self* (Farrar Straus Giroux).

Miller, A. (1988). *Banished Knowledge* (Farrar Straus Giroux).

Mrudula, G., Vrushabendra swamy, B.M. and Jayaveera, K.N. (2013). Evaluation of adaptogenic activity of Unani herb Borago officinalis, *Research & Reviews: Journal of Pharmacy and Pharmaceutical Sciences*. 2(2): 10–15.

Ogden, J. (2012). *Health Psychology A Textbook* (OUP).

Palmer, J.A., McCown, W. and Kerby, D. (1997). The adaptive significance of "dysfunctional" impulsivity. Paper presented at meeting of the Human Behavior and Evolution Society, Tucson, AR.

McCown, W., Palmer, J.A. and Thornburg, T. (1998). Impulsivity as an evolved conditional strategy. Paper presented at the meeting of the Human Behavior and Evolution Society, Davis, CA.

Priest, A.W. and Priest, L.R. (1983). *Herbal Medication: A Clinical and Dispensary Handbook* (Fowler).

Ross, J. (2010). *Combining Western hrbs and Chinese Medicine: A Clinical Materia Medica* (Verlag fur Ganzheitliche).

Sarno, J.E. (2010). *The Divided Mind: The Epidemic of Mindbody Disorders* (Duckworth Overlook).

Schienle, A., Stark R. and Vaitl D. (1998). Biological effects of incredibly low frequency (VLF) atmospherics in humans: a review. *J Sci Explor*, 12: 455–468.

Sinadinos, C., and Herbalist, C. (n.d.). 2018 *Herbal Therapeutic Treatments for Hypothyroidism*. Retrieved from https://www.americanherbalistsguild.com/sites/default/files/sinadinos_christa_-_herbal_support_for_hypothyroidism.pdf

Stableford, A. (2017). *Advanced Therapeutics lecture notes. BSc (Hons) Herbal Medicine* (Lincoln College).

Stout, J.H., Nicolai, M. and Sassovei, N. (2001). *The Human Lifebook* (Omniview Press).

Tafet, G.E., Idoyaga-Vargas, V.P., Abulafia, D.P. and Calandra J.M. (2001). Correlation between cortisol level and serotonin uptake in patients with chronic stress and depression. *Cognitive, Affective and Behavioural Neuroscience*, 1(4): 388–393.

Teeguarden, R. (1984). *Chinese Tonic Herbs* (Japan Publications).

Tirsch, W.S., Zenner, S., Ruhenstroth-Bauer, G. and Weinmann, H.M. (1994). Spektralanalytische Untersuchungen über den Einfluû der atmosphärischen Impulsstrahlung (Atmospherics) auf das menschliche EEG. (Spectroanalytical investigations about the influence of atmospherics on the human EEG). Abstract, EEG-Symposium Obergurgl, February 1994.

Tostes R.C., Nigro D., Z.B., Fortes Z.B. and Carvalho M.H.C. (2013). Effects of estrogen on the vascular system (Review). *Braz J Med Biol Res*, September 2003, 36(9): 1143–1158.

Vageto, E., Ciana, P. and Maggi, A. (2002). Estrogen and inflammation: hormone generous action spreads to the brain. *Molecular Psychiatry*, 7: 236–238.

Walter, S. 'Holistic as an Adjective not as a Noun' American Holistic Association. Ahha.org/scifhelp-articles (Accessed on August 14, 2019)

Weinhold, B. (2007). *The Flight From Intimacy: Healing Your Relationship of Counter-Dependence. The Other Side of Co-dependency* (New World Library).

Weinhold, B. and Weinhold, J. (2017). *Betrayal and the Path of the Heart* (CICRC Press).

Winnicott, D.W. (1960a). Ego distortion in terms of true and false self. In: *The Maturational Processes and the Facilitating Environment* (International Universities Press, 1987, pp. 140–152).

Winnicott, D.W. (1960b). The theory of the parent-infant relationship. In: *The Maturational Processes and the Facilitating Environment* (International Universities Press, 1987, pp. 233–225).

Wilson, J. (2001). *Adrenal Fatigue: The 21st Century Stress Syndrome* (Smart Publications).

Wilson, J. (2009). *Food Allergies, Sensitivities and Adrenal Fatigue* (The adrenal fatigue team). AdrenalFatigue.org.

Yance, D.R. (2013). *Adaptogens in Medical Herbalism* (Healing Arts Press).

Yehuda, R. and Bierer, L.M. (2009). The relevance of epigenetics to PTSD: Implications for the DSM-V. *J Trauma Stress*, 2009 Oct, 22(5): 427–434.

Further materials in support of this book, including photographs of tongues and conditions associated with the case histories, as well as additional case histories, can be found at the following website. This will also provide additional information about the author and his work and additional study opportunities.

https://www.andrewstableford.com

INDEX

Abulafia, D. P., 50
acne
    case history, 69
    vulgaris, 275. *See also* urticaria
ACTH. *See* adrenocorticotropic hormone
acute bacterial cystitis, remedy for, 219. *See also* urinary system
adaptogens, 128–131
Addison's disease, 110–111. *See also* fatigue
Adelson, E., 13
adrenal fatigue, 108. *See also* fatigue
    conditions associated with, 109
    indications of, 110
adrenal insufficiency, 108
adrenocorticotropic hormone (ACTH), 33
agrimonia, 135
AHHA. *See* American Holistic Health Association
American Holistic Health Association (AHHA), 6
amygdale, 50
Anderson, C. M., 240
ANS. *See* autonomic nervous system
anti-infective herbs, 209
anxiety, 141–142. *See also* nervous system
    case history, 152–154
    endometriosis, 233–234
Arndt-Schulz rule, 100
aromatase, 58
Aron, E., 24, 134

arthritis, 254, 256, 261–263. *See also* muscular-skeletal system
asteatotic, 273. *See also* skin disorders
atopic eczema, 272. *See also* skin disorders
autonomic nervous system (ANS), 2, 32
    balance, 9, 33–34
autonomic reactions, 29–32

Baldwin, A., 159
Barker, D., 13
    theory, 12–13
barking cough, 201. *See also* respiratory system
Bartram, T., 113
basal cell carcinomas, 276. *See also* urticaria
benign prostatic hypertrophy (BPH), 239, 242–243. *See also* male reproductive system
Betterle, C., 108
Bierer, L. M., 13
bisphenol-A (BPA), 240
Bjittebier, P., 24
blood
    deficiency, 38–39
    quality issues, 11
    tonification, 115
blood pressure, 54. *See also* clinical sign interpretation
    case history, 55–56
    diastolic, 56–57
    systolic, 56

body conscious, 19
Booth, C., 24
Boraginaceae, 84. *See also* herbs
Boutros, N. N., 25
BPA. *See* bisphenol-A
BPH. *See* benign prostatic hypertrophy
bradycardia, 59
Braun, C. A., 240
bronchial catarrh, 211–212. *See also* respiratory system
Bruining, H., 24
bullae, 271. *See also* lesions
bullous diseases, 275. *See also* urticaria
Butalid, L., 14
Bygren, L. O., 13

Calandra, J. M., 50
Cappola, A., 240
carcinoma, basal cell, 276. *See also* urticaria
cardiovascular disease, 56, 157
    case history, 168–169
cardiovascular index (CVI), 55–56
cardiovascular system, 157. *See also* cardiovascular disease
    case history, 166
    cerebral circulatory deficiency, 169–170
    circulatory herbs, 162–166
    haemorrhoids and varicose veins, 161
    heart, 157
    herbs for cardiovascular health, 159–160
    herbs for circulatory system, 162
    hyperglycaemia, 157
    hypertension, 157–158, 166–168
    insulin resistance syndrome, 159
    leg ulceration, 170–171
    metabolic syndrome, 158–159
    peripheral circulation, 159
    Raynaud's disease, 159
    venous system, 161
Carvalho, M. H. C., 58
case histories
    acne, 69
    anxiety, 152–154
    arthritis, 261–263
    benign prostatic hypertrophy, 242–243
    bronchial catarrh, 211–212
    cardiovascular disease, 168–169
    chronic cough, 210–211
    chronic sinus congestion, 73–74
    chronic urticaria, 279–280
    deficiency from fatigue, 132–137
    digestive complaint, 183–184
    digestive disturbance, 180–182
    disconnection, 78–80
    dysmenorrhoea, 234–235
    eczema, 281–282
    endometriosis, anxiety, 233–234
    enlarged right ventricle, 77–78
    fatigue, 131–132
    fibromyalgia, 258–261
    hepatitis, 196–198
    herpes simplex, 280–281
    hot flushes, 236
    hypertension, 74–77, 166–168
    hyperthyroidism, 250
    indigestion, 184–186
    infertility, 235–236
    irritable bladder, 218–219
    kidney stones, 219–220
    lichen planus, 277–278
    liver congestion, 198–199
    menopausal hot flushes, 238
    muscular or skeletal pains, 263–266
    obsessive-compulsive disorder, 154–156
    pain and inflammation, 266–267
    pompholyx eczema, 278–279
    pre-menstrual tension, 237
    primary hypothyroidism, 248–250
    prostate cancer 1, 243–244
    prostate cancer 2, 244–245
    respiratory case histories, 208–212
    rheumatoid arthritis, 71–72
    sore throat, 208–210
    stress, 80–81
    treatment rationale, 70–71
    uterine fibroids, 231–233
catarrh, 202. *See also* respiratory system
catecholamines, 50–51
Ceda, G., 240
central nervous system (CNS), 2
cerebral circulatory deficiency, 169–170. *See also* cardiovascular system
Ceresini, G., 240
Chinese medical terminology, 66
chronic. *See also* dermatology; fatigue; muscular-skeletal system; pruritic conditions; respiratory system
    cough, 210–211
    inflammatory conditions, 253
    plaque, 274

sinus congestion, 73–74
sodium-potassium imbalance, 110
urticaria, 279–280
chronic fatigue, 111. *See also* fatigue
    diet, 112–113
    exercise, 112
    sleep, 111
chronic kidney disease (CKD), 109, 213. *See also* urinary system
Ciana, P., 222
circulatory herbs, 162–166
clinical analysis and interpretation, 11–12
clinical sign interpretation, 53
    blood pressure, 54–56
    causes of sensorial experience of temperature, 63–67
    diastolic blood pressure, 56–57
    fever, 62–63
    hormone deficiency, 58
    hypothermia, 63
    immunological response, 58–59
    pulse, 59–62
    stress and tension, 57–58
    systolic blood pressure, 56
    temperature, 62
    tongue, 67–68
CNS. *See* central nervous system
congestion, 9–10, 39
conscience, 28–29
conscious, 28. *See also* integration psychology and neurobiology
consciousness, 19, 28
constitution, 8
constraint, 10, 33
context, 11
cortisol, 50, 254. *See also* muscular-skeletal system
cosmic two-by-four events, 20–21
Courvoisier's law, 188. *See also* liver
Cozolino, L., 23, 62
Cromwell, H. C., 25
crust, 272. *See also* lesions
CVI. *See* cardiovascular index
cytokines, 45

Daehnert, C., 19
deficiency, 9. *See also* fatigue
    nutritional, 66
    pattern, 108
    syndromes, 34
deficient response, 35

dehydroepiandrosterone (DHEA), 222. *See also* female reproductive system
Denissen, J. J. A., 14
depletion, 9, 108. *See also* fatigue
    factors, 32
depression, 142. *See also* nervous system
dermatitis herpetiformis, 275. *See also* urticaria
dermatology, 269
    acne vulgaris, 275
    asteatotic, 273
    atopic eczema, 272
    basal cell carcinomas, 276
    bullous diseases, 275
    case history, 277–282
    chronic plaque, 274
    chronic urticaria, 279–280
    classification of disorders, 272–273
    dermatitis herpetiformis, 275
    discoid, 273
    eczema, 272, 281–282
    hands, 273
    herbal therapeutic actions, 270–271
    herpes simplex, 280–281
    lesion terminology, 271–272
    lichen planus, 275, 277–278
    linear IgA disease, 275
    malignant melanoma, 276–277
    malignant skin tumours, 275
    nutrition, 270
    pityriasis rosea, 275
    pompholyx eczema, 278–279
    pruritic conditions, 273–274
    pruritis, 273–274
    psoriasis, 274
    rosacea, 275
    seborrheic, 273
    squamous cell carcinoma, 276
    urticaria, 274–277
    varicose, 273
De Vita, F., 240
DHEA. *See* dehydroepiandrosterone
DHT. *See* dihydro-testosterone
diastolic blood pressure, 56–57
differential diagnosis, 7–8
digestive system, 173
    autonomic regulation, 173–174
    case history, 180–182, 183
    disturbance, 110, 180–182, 183–184
    herb classification of, 176–177
    herbs for, 178–180

indigestion, 184–186
inflammation, 174
medicine composition, 182
medicine rationale, 182–183
dihydro-testosterone (DHT), 229. *See also* female reproductive system; male reproductive system
discoid, 273. *See also* skin disorders
disconnection, 78–80
dissociation, 11, 53
diuretics, 214. *See also* urinary system
Dobransky. P., 142
dopamine, 45
dosages, 99–100
dysmenorrhoea, 234–235. *See also* female reproductive system

eczema, 272, 281–282. *See also* skin disorders
   atopic, 272
   pompholyx, 278–279
ego, 17
egotism, 18, 23
electromagnetic fields (EMFs), 14
elemental influences, 14–15
embodiment, 11
EMFs. *See* electromagnetic fields
emotion, 95–96
emotional disharmony, 53
empirical egoism, 18
endocrine depletion, 36, 185
endometriosis, anxiety, 233–234. *See also* female reproductive system
energetic patterns, 40–43
energy
   depletion, 36–37
   foundation, 9
English tonics, 128–131
enlarged right ventricle, 77–78
epigenetics, 12–13
erosion, 272. *See also* lesions
erythema, 272. *See also* lesions
expectoration, 202. *See also* respiratory system
experience, 22

faith, 94
false
   fire, 188
   self, 19
fatigue, 107, 109
   adrenal, 108–109, 110
   blood tonification, 115
   case history, 131–137
   cellular metabolism, 113
   characteristics of Addison's, 110–111
   chronic sodium-potassium imbalance, 110
   circulation, 110
   classification of herbal actions, 113
   deficiency pattern, 108
   depletion, 108
   diet, 112–113
   digestive disturbances, 110
   emotional response, 111
   English tonics and adaptogens, 128–131
   exercise, 112
   gluten sensitivity and deficiency pattern, 134
   herbs for tonification, 116–127
   key signs and symptoms, 109
   libido, 110
   muscular aches, 109
   orthostatic hypotension test, 111
   overwhelmed, 109
   paradoxical pupillary reflex, 111
   psychological, 113
   sleep, 110, 111
   syndrome, 107, 248
   temperature, 110
   thinking patterns, 110
   tonics, 114, 115
   treatment for chronic, 111
Faust, V., 14
female reproductive system, 221
   case histories, 231–238
   constitutional dynamics, 222–223
   dehydroepiandrosterone, 222
   dysmenorrhoea, 234–235
   endometriosis, anxiety, 233–234
   herbs for, 224, 225–230
   hormone levels, 221
   hot flushes, 236, 238
   infertility, 235–236
   insufficient oestrogen, 222
   irritation, 221
   oestrogen dominance, 221
   pre-menstrual tension, 237
   relationship to other organ systems, 223
   testosterone, 222
   uterine fibroids, 231–233
Ferrucci, L., 240
fever, 62–63
fibromyalgia, 258–261. *See also* muscular-skeletal system
fire, 10

Fischer, T., 135
Fisichella, A., 240
flavor, 104–105
flower essences and development of higher self, 143
foetal imprinting, 13
Fogel, A., 254
follicle stimulating hormone (FSH), 236. *See also* female reproductive system
food additives, 222
formulae for treating children, 101. *See also* prescription
Fortes, Z. B., 58
Foucault, M., 21
foundation energy, 9
Fox, E., 24
Fraiberg, S., 13
FSH. *See* follicle stimulating hormone
functional illness, 8
fundamental energy state, 9

GABA, 45
gastrointestinal tract (GIT), 46
gating, 25
genitourinary tract (GUT), 191
Gerbershagen, H. U., 14
germ theory of disease, 13–14
ginseng, 135
GIT. *See* gastrointestinal tract
glossitis, 66
gluten sensitivity and deficiency pattern, 134
GnRH. *See* gonadotropin-releasing hormone
Gohil, K. J., 70, 259
gonadotropin-releasing hormone (GnRH), 45
Grave's disease, 247
Greven, C. U., 24
Gustafsson, J. A., 13
GUT. *See* genitourinary tract

haemorrhoids, 161. *See also* cardiovascular system
hands, 273. *See also* skin disorders
Hardt, J., 14
Hawkes, N., 134
head conscious, 19
heart, 157. *See also* cardiovascular system
heat, 10
Hempton, C-H., 135
hepatitis, 196–197. *See also* liver
hepatitis A, 197–198
herbal actions, 23, 143
    dermatology, 270–271
    fatigue, 113
    female reproductive system, 224
    liver, 190
    muscular-skeletal system, 255–256
    nervous system, 142
    respiratory system, 203–204
herbs, 3. *See also* prescription
    Boraginaceae, 84
    cardiovascular health, 159–160
    circulatory, 162–166
    classification for GI system, 176–177
    combinations of, 97
    contraindicated in pregnancy, 103
    development of higher self, 143
    digestive system, 178–180
    and emotional balance, 142–143
    energetic actions of, 143
    for integration and harmony, 83
    kidney function, 215–218
    Lamiaceae, 83–84
    liver function, 190–195
    medicinal formula, 99
    muscular-skeletal system, 257–258
    nervous system, 144–151
    qualities of, 97
    reproductive system, 225–230, 241–242
    respiratory system, 204–207
    rosacea, 83
    therapeutic movement and actions, 84–92
    therapeutics, 11
    tincture formulation, 197
    tonification, 116–127
Hering's law of cure, 12
herpes simplex, 280–281. *See also* dermatology
higher self, 143
highly sensitised person (HSP), 24
high sensory processing, 24
Hippocrates, 14
holistic medical systems, 5
Homberg, J., 24
hormesis, 100
hormone deficiency, 38, 58. *See also* clinical sign interpretation
hot flushes, 236. *See also* female reproductive system
HPA. *See* hypothalamic-pituitary-adrenal
HSP. *See* highly sensitised person
hyperglycaemia, 157. *See also* cardiovascular system
hypertension, 56, 157–158. *See also* cardiovascular system
    case history, 74–77, 166–168
hyperthyroidism, 247, 250. *See also* thyroid
hypoadrenia. *See* adrenal fatigue

hypotension, 56
hypothalamic-pituitary-adrenal (HPA), 45
hypothalamic-pituitary-gonadal axis, 45
hypothalamic-pituitary-thyroid axis, 45
hypothermia, 63
hypothyroidism, 247. *See also* thyroid

Idoyaga-Vargas, V. P., 50
illness, 2, 7, 142
    as behavioural construct, 96
    functional, 8
immunological response, 58–59. *See also* clinical sign interpretation
indigestion, 184–186
infertility, 235–236. *See also* female reproductive system
inflammation, 253. *See also* muscular-skeletal system
    chronic inflammatory conditions, 253
    factors associated with, 254–255
    factors to improve, 255
    pain and, 266–267
inflammatory cytokines, 240
insulin resistance syndrome, 159. *See also* cardiovascular system
integrated person, 17
    arousal regulation, 24
    consciousness, 19–20
    cosmic two-by-four' events, 20–21
    ego, 17
    egotism, 18, 23
    empirical egoism, 18
    experience, 22
    factors in integration and harmony, 18–23
    gating, 25
    head conscious and body conscious, 19
    herbal intervention, 23
    high sensory processing, 24
    limbic brain, 17
    observing ego, 21
    repressed pain, 20
    self-belief, 18
    sensitive person, 24–25
    sensitive vs. sensitised person, 24
    subconscious element, 17
    the self, 17
    transmarginal inhibition, 24
    true vs. false self, 19
    violet flower essence, 25
integration psychology and neurobiology, 27
    ANS balance, 33–34
    autonomic reactions and patterning, 29–32
    autonomic regulation and arousal, 31
    blood deficiency, 38–39
    catecholamines, 50–51
    causes of heat, 44
    congestion, 39
    conscious, 28
    cortisol action, 50
    deficiency syndromes, 34
    dopamine, 45
    energetic patterns, 32–33, 40–43
    energy depletion, 36–37
    excess syndromes, 37
    GABA, 45
    hormone deficiency, 38
    interactions, 45
    neurasthenia, 35
    neurotransmitter, 44–45, 46–50
    oestrogen, 45
    operation and control of organism, 27
    parasympathetic excess, 38
    progesterone, 45
    regulation mechanisms, 32
    re-patterning, 36
    resolution benefits, 36
    serotonin, 45
    shock, 36
    stress hormones, 45
    subconscious, 27–28
    super-conscious, 28
    sympathetic deficiency symptoms, 34–35
    testosterone, 45
    treatment protocols, 36
    unconscious, 27–28
irritable bladder, 218–219. *See also* urinary system

Janov, A., 13, 20
Jayaveera, K. N., 136

Kaati, G., 13
Kaminski, P., 25
Katkin, E. S., 8
Katz, R., 25
Kenner, D., 100
Kerby, D., 51
kidney stones, 219–220. *See also* urinary system
Kolb, B., 141
Kral, J. G., 13

Labiatae. See *Lamiaceae*
Lamiaceae (Labiatae), 83–84. *See also* herbs
Lauretani, F., 240
Law of Cure, 270. *See also* dermatology
leg ulceration, 170–171. *See also* cardiovascular system
lesions, 271–272. *See also* dermatology
leucoplakia, 66
LH. *See* luteinising hormone
libido, 239. *See also* male reproductive system
lichen. *See also* dermatology; lesions; urticaria
    planus, 275, 277–278
    simplex, 273
limbic brain, 17, 53
linear IgA disease, 275. *See also* urticaria
Lionetti, F., 24
liver, 187
    autonomic regulation, 187
    congestion, 188, 198–199
    control of liver physiology, 189
    Courvoisier's law, 188
    disharmony sources, 187–188
    heat, 201
    hepatitis case history, 196–198
    herbal action classifications, 190
    herbal tincture formulation, 197
    herbs for, 190–195
    inflammation, 188
    liver congestion, 198–199
    and other organ systems, 188–189
    therapeutic intervention, 189
Longmore, M., 159
Lowen, A., 18, 19, 20
luteinising hormone (LH), 45

Maciocia, G., 61
macule, 271. *See also* lesions
Maggi, A., 222
Maggio, M., 240
male reproductive system, 239
    benign prostatic hypertrophy, 242–243
    case history, 242–245
    herbs for, 241–242
    libido, 239
    metabolic syndrome, 240
    prostate cancer 1, 243–244
    prostate cancer 2, 244–245
    prostate hyperplasia, 239–241
malignant. *See also* urticaria
    melanoma, 276–277
    skin tumours, 275
MAO. *See* monoamine oxidase
Marrubium vulgare, 202
MC. *See* menstrual cycle
McCown, W., 51
Mears, R. P., 25
medical diagnosis, 7
melatonin, 32
menopausal hot flushes, 238. *See also* female reproductive system
menorrhagia, 234–235. *See also* female reproductive system
menstrual cycle (MC), 152
mental illness, 139. *See also* nervous system
    neurosis, 140
    personality disorder, 140–141
    psychosis, 140
    Rosenhan and Seligman's seven features, 139–140
    traditional classification, 140
metabolic syndrome, 158–159, 240. *See also* cardiovascular system
Mezzacappa, E. S., 8
Miller, A., 21, 23
Mitochondrial DNA, 113
monoamine oxidase (MAO), 45
morality, 32
Morlin, L., 108
Mrudula, G., 136
muscular-skeletal system, 253
    aches and pains, 263–266
    arthritis, 261–263
    case history, 258–267
    factors to improve inflammation, 255
    fibromyalgia, 258–261
    herbal actions, 255–256
    herbs for, 257–258
    inflammation factors, 254–255
    pain and inflammation, 266–267
    pathology, 256–257

negative emotion, 107
nervous system, 139
    anxiety, 141–142, 152–154
    case history, 152–156
    depression, 142
    energetic actions of herbs, 143
    herbal actions, 142
    herbal intervention classification, 143

    herbs for, 144–151
    herbs for harmony, 142–143
    higher self development, 143
    mental illness classification, 139
    neurosis, 140
    obsessive-compulsive disorder, 154–156
    personality disorder, 140–141
    psychosis, 140
    Rosenhan and Seligman's seven features, 139–140
    traditional classification, 140
    trophorestoratives, 142
neurasthenia, 35, 108–109, 142
neuroendocrine status, 9
neurosis, 140. *See also* nervous system
neurotransmitter, 46–50
    systems, 44–45
Nicolai, M., 18
Nigro, D. Z. B., 58
nodular prurigo, 273. *See also* lesions
nutritional deficiencies, 66

observing ego, 21
obsessive-compulsive disorder, 154–156. *See also* nervous system
oestrogen, 45, 58, 221. *See also* female reproductive system
    dominance, 221
    insufficient, 222
Ogden, J., 134
organ activation, 10
organ energy potential, 10
organic illness, 8
orthodox medicine, 1
orthostatic hypotension test, 111. *See also* fatigue
osteoarthritis, 253. *See also* muscular-skeletal system
osteoporosis, 256–257. *See also* muscular-skeletal system

pain, repressed, 20
Palmer, J. A., 51
Palmer, S. N., 8
papule, 271. *See also* lesions
paradoxical pupillary reflex, 111. *See also* fatigue
parasympathetic excess, 38
pathogenic factors, 13–14
pathophysiology, 1
patterning, 29–32. *See also* integration psychology and neurobiology
PCOS. *See* polycystic ovarian syndrome
Penke, L., 14

peripheral circulation, 159. *See also* cardiovascular system
personality disorder, 140–141. *See also* nervous system
personal strengths, 22
phlegm, 202. *See also* respiratory system
physiology, 11
pityriasis rosea, 275. *See also* urticaria
plaque, 271. *See also* lesions
Pluess, M., 24
polycystic ovarian syndrome (PCOS), 69, 228. *See also* female reproductive system
pompholyx eczema, 278–279. *See also* dermatology
potential energy, 8
pre-menstrual tension, 237. *See also* female reproductive system
prescription, 93
    active vs. passive engagement of patient, 94–95
    Arndt-Schulz rule or Schulz' law, 100
    dosages, 99–100
    emotion, 95–96
    factors for prescribing, 97
    formulae for treating children, 101
    herbal medicine formula, 99
    herb combinations, 97
    herbs contraindicated in pregnancy, 103
    hormesis, 100
    illness as behavioural construct, 96
    intention, 93–94
    qualities of flavor, 104–105
    qualities of herbs, 97
    reassurance vs. self-actualisation, 95
    science of prescribing, 94
    self-belief, 94
    sensorial impact, 96–97
    triads, 98
    unexpected outcomes and defence reactions, 101–102
Priest, A. W., 54
Priest, L. R., 54
primary hypothyroidism, 248–250. *See also* thyroid
progesterone, 45
prostate. *See also* male reproductive system
    cancer 1, 243–244
    cancer 2, 244–245
    hyperplasia, 239–241
prostate-specific antigen (PSA), 242
prostatic hypertrophy, benign, 239, 242–243. *See also* male reproductive system
Prunus serorinta, 202

pruritic conditions, 273. *See also* dermatology
    chronic plaque, 274
    pruritis, 273–274
    psoriasis, 274
PSA. *See* prostate-specific antigen
psoriasis, 274. *See also* pruritic conditions
psychology, 11
psychosis, 140. *See also* nervous system
pulse, 59–60. *See also* clinical sign interpretation
    characteristics, 60
    Chinese patterns, 61
    depth of, 60
    diagnosis, 60
    factors affecting, 60
    right vs. left, 62
pustule, 271. *See also* lesions

Qi, 66

Raynaud's disease, 64, 159. *See also* cardiovascular system
realised energy, 8
re-patterning, 36
repressed pain, 20
Requena, Y., 100
resolution, 36
respiratory system, 201
    autonomic regulation, 201
    barking cough, 201
    bronchial catarrh, 211–212
    case histories, 208–212
    catarrh, 202
    chronic cough, 210–211
    expectoration, 202
    herb classification, 203–204
    herbs for, 204–207
    inflammation, 201–202
    liver heat, 201
    Marrubium vulgare, 202
    phlegm, 202
    Prunus serorinta, 202
    rising liver heat issue, 209
    sore throat, 208–210
    therapeutic intervention, 202
reverse T3 (rT3), 45
rheumatoid arthritis, 253. *See also* muscular-skeletal system
    case history, 71–72
rising liver heat, 188
    issue, 209

ritual, 30
rosacea, 83, 275. *See also* herbs; urticaria
Rosenhan and Seligman's seven features, 139–140
Rosmarinus, 186
Ross, J., 241, 242
rT3. *See* reverse T3
Ruhenstroth-Bauer, G., 15

Sarno, J. E., 20
Sassovei, N., 18
scale, 272. *See also* lesions
Schienle, A., 15
Schnedan, H. E., 24
Schulz' law, 100
Schumann resonance, 15
sclerosis, 272. *See also* lesions
seborrheic, 273. *See also* skin disorders
selective serotonin reuptake inhibitors (SSRIs), 51
self, the, 17
    -belief, 94
    higher, 143
    sense of, 2
    true, 19
sense of
    agency, 23
    self, 2
sensorial experience of temperature, 63. *See also* clinical sign interpretation
    cold, 63–64
    cold feet, 64
    facial colour, 65
    heat, 64–65
    important distinctions, 66
    respiration, 65
    tongue diagnosis, 65–66
    tongue examination, 66–67
sensorial impact, 96–97
Serenoa, 239
serotonin, 32, 45
sex hormone binding globulin (SHBG), 189
sferics, 14
Shapiro, V., 13
SHBG. *See* sex hormone binding globulin
shock, 36
skin disorders, 272. *See also* dermatology
    asteatotic, 273
    atopic eczema, 272
    discoid, 273
    eczema, 272
    hands, 273

seborrheic, 273
venous/varicose, 273
skin pathology, 269–270. *See also* dermatology
smooth muscle tone, 33
sore throat, 208–210. *See also* respiratory system
spiritual pride, 23
squamous cell carcinoma, 276. *See also* urticaria
SSRIs. *See* selective serotonin reuptake inhibitors
Stableford, A., 134, 136
Stark, R., 15
steroidal hormones, 58
Stout, J. H., 18
stress. *See also* clinical sign interpretation
   case history, 80–81
   hormones, 45
   and tension, 57–58
subconscious, 27–28. *See also* integration psychology and neurobiology
subtle communication, 28
super-conscious, 28, 29. *See also* integration psychology and neurobiology
sympathetic
   deficiency, 34–35
   system, 33
   tone, 11
symptoms, 12
systolic, 56
systolic blood pressure, 56

tachycardia, 59
tachypnoea, 65
Tafet, G. E., 50
Taoism, 5
Tao, The, 5
Teeguarden, R., 135
temperature, 62
testosterone, 45, 222. *See also* female reproductive system
therapeutic
   intervention, 15
   principles, 7–15
thyroid, 247
   case history, 248–250
   fatigue syndrome, 248
   Grave's disease, 247
   hyperthyroidism, 247, 250
   hypothyroidism, 247, 248–250
   nutrition, 248
   treatment protocols, 248

Ticinesi, A., 240
Tirsch, W. S., 15
tongue, 67. *See also* clinical sign interpretation
   coating, 68
   colour of body, 67
   cracking, 68
   moisture, 68
   shape, 67–68
   spirit or vitality, 67
tonics, 114
   and adaptogens, 128–131
   formulations, 115
tonification
   blood, 115
   herbs for, 116–127
Tostes, R. C., 58
transgenerational transmission of stress, 13
transmarginal inhibition, 24
treatment
   protocols, 248
   rationale, 70–71
triads, 98
trophorestoratives, 142
true self, 19

ulcer, 272. *See also* lesions
unconscious, 27–28. *See also* integration psychology and neurobiology
urinary system, 213
   case history, 218–220
   causative factors, 213
   cystitis treatment, 219
   diuretics, 214
   herbs for kidney function, 215–218
   irritable bladder, 218–219
   kidney stones, 219–220
urtica, 272. *See also* lesions
urticaria, 57–58, 274. *See also* dermatology
   acne vulgaris, 275
   basal cell carcinomas, 276
   bullous diseases, 275
   dermatitis herpetiformis, 275
   lichen planus, 275
   linear IgA disease, 275
   malignant melanoma, 276–277
   malignant skin tumours, 275
   pityriasis rosea, 275
   rosacea, 275

squamous cell carcinoma, 276
uterine fibroids, 231–233. *See also* female reproductive system

Vageto, E., 222
Vaitl, D., 15
van Aken, M. A. G., 14
varicose veins, 161, 273. *See also* cardiovascular system
venous system, 161. *See also* cardiovascular system
very-low-frequency (VLF), 14
vesicle, 271. *See also* lesions
vital
    force, 5–6
    function of individual, 9
    person, 5
VLF. *See* very-low-frequency
Vrushabendra swamy, B. M., 136

Wallin, E., 159
Walter, S., 6
Wan, L., 25
Wehner, W., 14
Weidmann, M., 14
Weinhold, B., 21, 22
Weinhold, J., 21
Weinmann, H. M., 15
Western
    herbal medicine, 1
    medical diagnosis, 7–8
    medical terminology, 7
Whishaw, I., 141
Wilkinson, I. B., 159
Wilson, J., 59, 134
Winnicott, D. W., 19, 21
Wyrd, 2

Yance, D. R., 241, 242
Yehuda, R., 13

Zenner, S., 15

www.ingramcontent.com/pod-product-compliance
Ingram Content Group UK Ltd.
Pitfield, Milton Keynes, MK11 3LW, UK
UKHW060153230226
468275UK00010B/154